Outline of Clinical Diagnosis in the Goat

To my wife Hilary who understands goats
and my mother Lesley who never will

Outline of Clinical Diagnosis in the Goat

John G. Matthews BSc, BVMS, MRCVS
Clarendon House Veterinary Centre,
Chelmsford, UK

WRIGHT
London   Boston   Singapore   Sydney   Toronto   Wellington

Wright
An imprint of Butterworth–Heinemann Ltd.,
Halley Court, Jordan Hill, Oxford OX2 8EJ

 PART OF REED INTERNATIONAL P.L.C.

OXFORD   LONDON   GUILDFORD   BOSTON   MUNICH
NEW DELHI   SINGAPORE   SYDNEY   TOKYO
TORONTO   WELLINGTON

First published 1991

© Butterworth–Heinemann Ltd., 1991

British Library Cataloguing in Publication Data
Matthews, John G.
   Outline of clinical diagnosis in the goat.
   1. Livestock goats diagnosis
   I. Title
   ISBN 0-7236-1475-X

Library of Congress Cataloging in Publication Data
Matthews, John G.
   Outline of clinical diagnosis in the goat/John G. Matthews.
      p.   cm.
   Includes bibliographical references and index.
   ISBN 0-7236-1475-X:
   1. Goats – Diseases – Diagnosis. 2. Veterinary clinical pathology
   I. Title.
   SF968.M37   1991
   636.3′9089′6075 – dc20

Text processed by David Coates, Tunbridge Wells, Kent
Photosetting and composition by Genesis Typesetting, Laser Quay,
Rochester, Kent
Printed and bound in Great Britain by Courier International Ltd., Tiptree, Essex

Preface

The increasing interest in goats in the UK, both for milk and fibre production, has been matched by a corresponding awareness in the veterinary profession that the species merits consideration as an animal in its own right. The formation of the Goat Veterinary Society in 1979 provided a means of collating and disseminating information on goat management and disease control but until now there has been no readily available text covering goat diseases. Hopefully this book will, at least in part, fill that gap.

The book gives an outline of the more common clinical problems likely to be met by the general practitioner involved with goat medicine, with each chapter covering a major presenting sign. Each chapter starts with the initial assessment and clinical examination of the patient, together with further investigations, which may aid diagnosis, before considering specific diseases, their diagnosis, clinical signs and treatment. At the end of each chapter there is a short list of references – these are generally review articles which the clinician will find of interest. A list of general references is included at the end of the book. In addition there is a chapter on Plant Poisoning.

It has been said that the goat is 'mostly sheep and partly cow' and, undoubtedly, any veterinary surgeon with a working knowledge of other ruminants should be able satisfactorily to diagnose and treat most medical conditions in the goat. There are, however, important behavioural and physiological differences between the species resulting, in many instances, in important differences in their response to disease, so that it is not always safe to extrapolate from one species to another. In addition, drug metabolism shows species variation with the result that dose rates and excretion times for goats are not simply obtained from cow or sheep data. I hope that having read this book, the clinician will feel confident in treating not a small cow or a large milking sheep but the animal in its own right – the goat.

Acknowledgements

I acknowledge with grateful thanks the forbearance of my colleagues at Clarendon House Veterinary Centre during the writing of this book and in particular thank Mrs Janice Bromley for painstakingly typing the manuscript.

My wife Hilary has provided encouragement and support and given valuable advice on goat husbandry.

Author's note

For many medical conditions, there are no drugs available which are specifically licensed for goats. Dose rates are quoted in the book for many unlicensed drugs. These dose rates have been obtained from published reports, data held on file by the drug manufacturers and from personal experience. Wherever possible, the clinician should use drugs which carry a full product licence for caprine treatment. If in doubt about the use or dosage of any drug, consult the manufacturer. In all cases where unlicensed drugs are used, milk should not be used for human consumption for 7 days and meat for 28 days following the administration of the drug.

Contents

1 Female infertility

The investigation of female infertility
Pregnancy diagnosis
Use of prostaglandins

The investigation of female infertility

The investigation of female infertility in the goat presents major
difficulties when compared with that in the cow because of the
inability to palpate the ovaries and because of the seasonal
pattern of breeding – does are often presented towards the end
of the season, limiting the time available for remedial measures
(Table 1.1).

Preliminary history

Consider:

- Individual or flock/herd problem.
- Feeding, including mineral supplementation.
- Management practices – handmating, artificial insemination
  (AI), buck running with does.
- Disease status of herd/flock.
  If there is a *herd problem* (Table 1.2), investigate:
- Male infertility (qv).
- Intercurrent disease – parasitism, footrot etc.
- Nutritional status – energy or protein deficit, mineral
  deficiency (phosphorus, copper, iodine, manganese).
- Stress – overcrowding, recent grouping of goats.
- Poor heat detection.
- Services at incorrect time.

Assessment of individual doe

(1) General assessment
   Conformation
   Body condition
   Dentition
   Clinical examination

Any obvious clinical signs such as debility, anaemia or
lameness should be investigated and corrected where possible
before commencing specific therapy aimed at correcting a
reproductive disorder.

In the UK overfeeding is probably a greater cause of infertility
than poor condition.

(2) Specific examination of the reproductive and mammary
   systems. Include, where necessary, examination of the
   vagina and cervix with a speculum to identify anatomical
   abnormalities.

Table 1.1

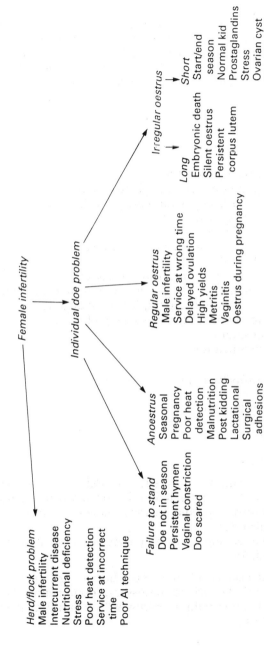

Female infertility

Herd/flock problem
Male infertility
Intercurrent disease
Nutritional deficiency
Stress
Poor heat detection
Service at incorrect
time
Poor AI technique

Individual doe problem

Failure to stand
Doe not in season
Persistent hymen
Vaginal constriction
Doe scared

Anoestrus
Seasonal
Pregnancy
Poor heat
detection
Malnutrition
Post kidding
Lactational
Surgical
adhesions
Hydrometra
Intersex
Freemartin
Ovarian malfunction

Regular oestrus
Male infertility
Service at wrong time
Delayed ovulation
High yields
Metritis
Vaginitis
Oestrus during pregnancy

Irregular oestrus

Long
Embryonic death
Silent oestrus
Persistent
corpus lutem

Short
Start/end
season
Normal kid
Prostaglandins
Stress
Ovarian cyst
Metritis
Mummified kid

Table 1.2 Causes of herd/flock problems of infertility

Male infertility
Intercurrent disease
Nutritional deficiency
Stress
Poor heat detection
Service at incorrect time
Poor AI technique

---

(3) *Specific history*
- Date of last kidding/stage of lactation.
- Daily milk yield.
- Presence or absence of obvious oestrus signs.
- Length of oestrus cycles.
- Date of last service.
- Willingness to stand for male.
- Kidding difficulties last time – malpresentation/ manipulation, metritis, retained placenta, abortion, mummified fetus, still births.

(4) *Further investigations*
- Specific laboratory tests
  progesterone assay
  oestrone sulphate assay
  bacteriological examination of vaginal or uterine samples
  feed analysis
- Laparoscopy or laparotomy
- Realtime ultrasound scanning

Individual infertility problems will generally fall into one of four categories.

(a) Difficulty at service
(b) Anoestrus
(c) Regular oestrus
(d) Irregular oestrus

(a) *Difficulty at service*

- Doe not in season.
- Doe scared – common with maiden animals, particularly if a large buck is used on a small doe.
- Persistent hymen or vaginal constriction.

Table 1.3 Causes of anoestrus

Seasonal
Pregnancy
Poor heat detection
Malnutrition
Post kidding anoestrus
Lactational anoestrus
Adhesions following surgery
Hydrometra
Intersex
Freemartin
Ovarian malfunction

(b) Anoestrus (Table 1.3)

- *Seasonal* – most goats are totally anoestrus in the northern hemisphere between March and August, although fertile matings have been recorded in all months of the year. Anglo Nubian goats in particular have extremely long breeding seasons. Recently imported animals from the southern hemisphere may take time to adjust to a new seasonality. The breeding season is initiated largely in response to decreasing day length, but is also dependent on temperature, the environment (particularly nutrition) and the presence of a male. Decreasing day length also stimulates reproductive activity in the buck.
- *Pregnancy* – the possibility of an undetected pregnancy should *always* be considered (even if the owner insists that no mating has occurred) before attempting treatment, particularly with prostaglandins.
- *Poor heat detection* – although some dairy does show only minor behavioural changes during oestrus, *oestrus detection* is generally easier than in Angora goats, most does showing obvious signs of tail wagging, frequent bleating, urination near the buck, swelling of the vulva and a mucous vaginal discharge. The signs are generally accentuated in the presence of a male or even a 'billy rag' i.e. a cloth which has been rubbed on the head of the buck and stored in a sealed jar.

Oestrus can be determined visually by means of a speculum. At the onset of heat the cervix changes from its normal white colour becoming hyperaemic and the cervical secretions are thin and clear. The secretions rapidly thicken, becoming grey/white and collecting on the floor of the vagina.

Unlike cows most does will not stand to be ridden by other females even when in oestrus. Riding behaviour is sometimes seen as an expression of dominance in the herd or as part of the nymphomaniac behaviour of goats with cystic ovaries.

Many young bucks will mount and serve females which are not in true standing oestrus if the female is restrained, although older bucks are usually more discriminating. The doe will stand to be mated only when she is in oestrus.

In the milking doe, a rise in milk production may occur 8–12 hours before the start of oestrus and milk production may fall below normal during oestrus.

When the buck is running with the flock or herd, sire harnesses with raddles or marker paste will aid oestrus detection. A marked vasectomized ('teaser') buck can be used to detect (and help initiate) the start of oestrus in a group of does.

- *Malnutrition* – An energy or protein deficit due either to poor nutrition or intercurrent disease may cause anoestrus.
  Deficiencies of minerals such as cobalt, selenium, manganese, zinc, phosphorus, iodine and copper and deficiencies of vitamins B_{12} and D are all reported to cause infertility.
- *Postkidding anoestrus* – Many does will not show signs of oestrus for 3 months or more after kidding even if kidding takes place during the normal breeding season.
- *Lactational anoestrus* – Some high yielding does do not exhibit marked signs of oestrus. These animals may respond to prostaglandin injections with careful observation for oestrus 24–48 hours later. Animals which do not respond may need a further injection 11 days later.
- *Adhesions following surgery* – The goat's reproductive tract is sensitive to handling and adhesions will occur unless very high standards of surgery are maintained during embryo transplant or other surgical procedures. Talc from surgical gloves will produce a marked tissue reaction.
- *Hydrometra (pseudopregnancy, cloudburst)* – Hydrometra is defined as a pathological condition of the uterus in which accumulation of aseptic fluid takes place in the presence of a persistent corpus luteum, which continues to secrete progesterone.

Aetiology:
(1) a persistent corpus luteum following an oestrus cycle in which pregnancy did not occur. This is common in goats

which are running through and not mated. Certain families seem prone to develop the condition.

(2) a persistent corpus luteum following embryonic death with resorption of the embryo.

Clinical signs: the doe acts as if pregnant with enlargement of the abdomen and a degree of udder development if not milking. Milking does may show a sharp drop in yield and this may result in a significant economic loss if the condition is not corrected. Fetal fluids collect in the abdomen and the doe may become enormously distended.

When the hydrometra occurs following embryonic death the pseudopregnancy generally persists for the full gestational length or longer before luteolysis occurs, progesterone secretion ceases and the fetal fluids are released ('cloudburst'). Some does milk adequately following the cloudburst.

When the hydrometra occurs in a doe which has not been mated, the release of fluids often occurs in less than the normal gestation period, the doe may cycle again and a further hydrometra occur. Subsequent pregnancies are not generally affected but the doe is likely to develop the condition again in the following year.

If the hydrometra follows fetal death, fetal membranes and possibly a decomposed fetus are present, otherwise no fetal membranes are formed.

Diagnosis:
(1) realtime ultrasound scanning of the right ventrolateral abdominal wall shows large fluid compartments. Scanning should take place at least 40 days after mating to avoid confusion with early pregnancy.
(2) elevated milk or plasma progesterone levels consistent with pregnancy, but low milk or plasma oestrone sulphate levels.
(3) X-ray fails to show fetal skeletons in an anoestrus doe with a distended abdomen.

Treatment: prostaglandin injection. It is possible that Lutalyse (UpJohn) which has a direct effect on uterine muscle is preferable to Estrumate (Coopers Pitman-Moore) in treating hydrometra.

An oxytocin injection (15 i.u.) a few days after treatment with prostaglandin stimulates uterine contractions and aids involution.

- *Intersex (pseudohermaphrodite)* – In goats the dominant gene for polledness is associated with a recessive gene for intersex. Intersex is a recessive sex linked incompletely penetrant trait resulting from the breeding of two polled goats.

  A mating between a homozygous (PP) polled male and a heterozygous (Pp) polled female will produce 50% intersexes; a mating between a heterozygous (Pp) polled male and a heterozygous (Pp) polled female will produce 25% intersexes.

  Affected animals are genetically female with a normal female chromosome complement (60 XX), but phenotypically show great variation from phenotypic male to phenotypic female. Some animals are obviously abnormal at birth with a normal vulva but enlarged clitoris or a penile clitoris. The gonads are generally testes which may be abdominal or scrotal and phenotypic males may have a shortened penis (hypospadias), hypoplastic testes, or sperm granuloma in the head of the epididymis. Other animals may reach maturity before being detected and may present as being anoestrus. A phenotypically female animal may have male characteristics due to internal testes.

- *Freemartins* – The freemartin condition with hypoplasia of the female gonads and XX/XY chimaerism occurs occasionally in female goats which are born cotwin to males, following vascular anastomosis in early gestation.
- *Ovarian malfunction* – Ovarian inactivity is poorly understood in the goat but some anoestrus goats will respond to treatment with gonadotrophin releasing hormones (Receptal, Hoechst) – use cow doses. Other goats will respond to treatment with prostaglandins suggesting a retained corpus luteum or luteinized cystic ovaries. Increased use of laparoscopic techniques may aid the diagnosis of these conditions

(c) Irregular oestrus cycles (Table 1.4)

- *Long oestrus cycles*
  - (1) *Embryonic death* – Early embryonic death with loss of the corpus luteum will produce a subsequent return to oestrus following resorption of the embryonic material. Following embryonic death, a percentage of does will not return to oestrus but develop hydrometra.
  - (2) *Silent oestrus* – Some does will exhibit oestrus early in the season and then show no further oestrus signs for some

Table 1.4 Irregular oestrus cycles

Long	Short
Embryonic death	Start/end of season
Silent oestrus	Normal kid behaviour
Persistent corpus luteum	Prostaglandins
	Stress
	Ovarian follicular cyst
	Metritis
	Mummified kid

months. These goats may be cycling silently and will respond to treatment with prostaglandins.

(3) *Persistent corpus luteum* – Failure of the corpus luteum to undergo luteolysis at the correct time will delay the return to oestrus.

- *Short oestrus cycles (less than 18–21 days)*
  (i) Short anovulatory cycles of about 7 days are common at the start of the breeding season and occasionally occur at the end of the breeding season.
  (ii) Kids commonly show short cycles during their first breeding season.
  (iii) Very short oestrus cycles have been recorded following administration of prostaglandins to abort does. A normal oestrus pattern returns after 3–4 weeks.
  (iv) Premature regression of the corpus luteum is recognized as a problem in goats undergoing oestrus synchronization for embryo transplant. In some cases this will be a result of stress (see below). In other cases, the cause is unknown.
  (v) Groups of goats which are stressed will often show short cycles of around 7 days presumably because of premature regression of the corpus luteum. For this reason goats being brought together for a breeding programme, e.g. for embryo transplant should be grouped at least 3 months before the start of the programme.
  (vi) Ovarian follicular cysts produce oestrogens which result in a shortened oestrus cycle of between 3 and 7 days or continuous heat. Eventually the oestrogenic effects produce relaxed pelvic ligaments and the goat

displays male-like mounting behaviour. The diagnosis can be confirmed by laparoscopy or laparotomy.

Medical treatment with chorionic gonadotrophin (Chorulon 1000 i.u. i.m., Intervet) or gonadotrophin releasing hormones (Receptal 5.0 ml i.m., Hoechst) is only successful if commenced early. Surgical treatment to exteriorize and rupture the thick wall of the cyst should be considered in valuable animals.

(vii) Endometritis may cause short cycling or return to oestrus at the normal time.

(viii) Vaginitis – see regular oestrus cycles.

(ix) The presence of fetal bone remaining from a mummified kid which is not expelled at parturition will act as a constant source of stimulation and result in short oestrus cycles. There may be a history of bones and fetal material being expelled at kidding or subsequently.

(d) Regular oestrus cycles (Table 1.5)

- *Male infertility* (qv).
- *Service at the wrong time.*
- *Delayed ovulation/follicular atresia.*

There is little scientific evidence describing these conditions in goats but in practice a 'holding' injection of chorionic gonadotrophin, 500 i.u. Chorulon (Intervet) or gonadotrophin releasing hormones 2.5 ml i.m. Receptal (Hoechst) given at the time of service or AI will aid fertility in some animals by stimulating ovulation on the day of service.

- *High yielding females* – Some high yielding females may have suboptimum fertility possibly due to a pituitary dysfunction resulting from the heavy lactation. Chorionic gonadotrophin (500 i.u. Chorulon, Intervet) may promote

Table 1.5 Regular oestrus cycles

Male infertility
Service at wrong time
Delayed ovulation
High yielders
Metritis
Vaginitis
Oestrus during pregnancy

maturation of follicles, ovulation and formation of the corpus luteum.

- *Metritis* – A low grade metritis may result in the failure of the embryo to implant and subsequent return to service at the normal time.
- *Vaginitis* – occasionally occurs, particularly after the removal of vaginal sponges. Vaginitis may result in short oestrus cycles or repeated return to service at a normal cycle length.

   In New Zealand and Australia, caprine herpes virus type 1 causes vulvovaginitis with short oestrus cycles.

- *Oestrus during pregnancy* – A few goats exhibit regular oestrus signs during pregnancy although this is less common than in cattle. Ovulation does not occur and the signs of oestrus are usually rather weak. Accurate pregnancy diagnosis is important before attempting treatment, particularly with prostaglandins

Pregnancy diagnosis

Non-return to service is *not* a reliable method of pregnancy diagnosis. Some does may not outwardly cycle throughout the breeding season, the incidence of false pregnancies is fairly high particularly in some strains of dairy goats and if the service was at the end of the breeding season non-return may be due to seasonal anoestrus. Similarly *mammary development* in primaparous goats is *not* a reliable indicator of pregnancy.

(1) Oestrone sulphate assay

Oestrone sulphate concentrations in milk and plasma increase steadily during pregnancy and can be used to diagnose pregnancy 50 days post service.

   Milk or blood samples can be submitted to the Milk Marketing Board (MMB, Veterinary Laboratory, Cleeve House, Lower Wick, Worcester WR2 4NS) and some other commercial laboratories.

   This test will distinguish between true pregnancy and hydrometra, but occasional false negatives do occur particularly if the sampling is close to 50 days and repeat sampling may be indicated before the induction of oestrus with prostaglandins to avoid the possibility of aborting a pregnant doe.

(2) Ultrasonic scanning

Realtime ultrasonic scanning has the added advantage of giving *some* indication of the number of kids being carried thus enabling a better estimate of the nutritional requirements of the doe during pregnancy. The technique is virtually 100% accurate in determining pregnancy and 96–97% accurate in determining twins and triplets. Good operators can distinguish hydrometra and resorbed fetuses as well as live kids.

Scanning can be used from 28 days post service when a fluid filled uterus can be identified but is best used between 50 and 100 days of pregnancy. Cotyledons can be distinguished from about 40 days, individual fetuses by 45–50 days. By 100 days individual fetuses more than fill the entire screen making accurate determination of numbers difficult.

(3) Doppler ultrasound techniques

Doppler ultrasound techniques can detect the fetal pulse after about 2 months' gestation, using either an intrapelvic probe or an external probe placed on a clipped site immediately in from the right udder or lateral to the left udder using vegetable oil to improve contact.

Between 60 and 120 days' gestation the accuracy in detecting non-pregnancy is more than 90% but the method is unreliable in detecting multiple fetuses.

Other methods are sometimes useful:

(4) Progesterone assay

Progesterone secreted by the corpus luteum of a pregnant goat can be detected by radioimmunoassay or by ELISA methods in milk or in plasma. Progesterone levels remain high throughout pregnancy.

Random sampling will not lead to accurate pregnancy diagnosis because the corpus luteum of the normal oestrus cycle and that of hydrometra also produce progesterone. A sample taken 24 days after mating will give nearly 100% accuracy in determining non-pregnancy but only about 85–90% accuracy in determining pregnancy because of factors such as early embryonic death and hydrometra. A low progesterone level always indicates non-pregnancy.

(5) X-ray

Fetal skeletons are detectable between 70 and 80 days although the technique is more useful after 90 days.
An enlarged uterus may be detected at 38 days and over.

(6) Rectoabdominal palpation

In the non-pregnant goat a plastic rod inserted in the rectum can be palpated at the body wall. Between 70 and 100 days post service, the pregnant uterus prevents palpation of the rod. The technique produces unacceptably high levels of fetal mortality and risk of rectal perforation.

(7) Ballotment

Ballotment of the right flank or ventrally is a time honoured goat keepers' technique for pregnancy diagnosis but in the author's experience is extremely unreliable. Fetal movements can often be observed in the right flank of the doe during the last 30 days of gestation.

Use of prostaglandins

Unlike other ruminants where placenta-derived progesterone becomes significant, the goat depends on corpus-luteum-derived progesterone throughout pregnancy, and is thus susceptible to luteolytic agents, including prostaglandins, throughout the whole of pregnancy.
Prostaglandins can be used for:

- Timing of oestrus
- Synchronization of oestrus
- Misalliance
- Abortion
- Timing and synchronization of parturition
- Treatment of hydrometra
- Treatment of persistent corpus luteum

Recommended doses of prostaglandins in dairy goats are 0.5 ml Estrumate (Coopers Pitman-Moore) or 2 ml Lutalyse (Upjohn). Smaller doses will produce luteolysis in Angora

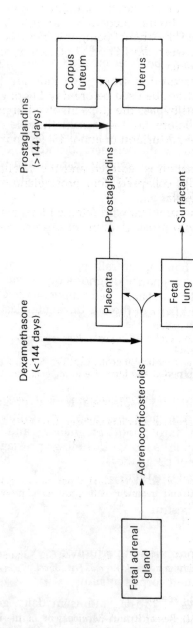

Figure 1.1 Induction of parturition

goats. The effect of prostaglandin administration, is seen between 24 and 48 hours (generally around 36 hours) postinjection, provided the animal being injected has an active corpus luteum, i.e. between days 4 and 17 of the normal oestrus cycle or during pregnancy.

For induction of parturition where live kids are required, prostaglandins should not be used before day 144 of gestation, because prostaglandins bypass the steps involved in producing fetal lung surfactant. Before day 144, dexamethasone should be used and will produce parturition in about 48–96 hours (Figure 1.1).

Where rapid termination is required and the viability of the kids is not critical, e.g. collapsed doe, prostaglandins can be used at any stage of gestation.

There is generally no problem with retained fetal membranes following induction with prostaglandins or dexamethasone.

Further Reading

General

Evans, G. and Maxwell, W. M. C. (1987) *Salamon's Artificial Insemination of Sheep and Goats*, Butterworths, London

Howe, P. A. (1984) Breeding problems in goats. *Proc. Univ. Sydney Post Grad Comm. Vet. Sci.*, **73**, 511–514

Mews, A. (1981) Breeding and fertility in goats. *Goat Vet. Soc. J.*, **2** (2), 2–11

Peaker, M. (1978) Gestation period and litter size in the goat. *Bri. Vet. J.*, **134**, 379–383

Skelton, M. (1978) Reproduction and breeding of goats. *J. Dairy Science*, **61**, 994–1010

Ward, W. R. (1980) Some aspects of infertility in the goat. *Goat Vet. Soc. J.*, **1** (2), 2–5

Hydrometra

Pieterse, M. C. and Taverne, M. A. M. (1986) Hydrometra in goats: diagnosis with realtime ultrasound and treatment with prostaglandins or oxytocin. *Theriogenology*, **26**, 813–821

Intersexes

Hamerton, J. L., Dickson, J. M., Pollard, C. E., Grieves, S. A. and Short, R. V. (1969) Genetic intersexuality in goats. *J. Reprod. Fert. Suppl.*, **7**, 25–51

Control of the breeding season

Corteel, J. M. *et al.* (1982) Research and development in the control of reproduction. In *Proceedings III International Conference on Goat Production and Disease*, 584–591

Geary, M. R. (1982) Use of Chronogest sponges and PMSG. *Goat Vet. Soc. J.*, **3** (2), 5–6

Henderson, D. C. (1985) Control of the breeding season in sheep and goats. *In Practice*, July 1985, 118–123

Henderson, D. C. (1987) Manipulation of the breeding season in goats – a review. *Goat Vet. Soc. J.*, **8** (1), 7–16

Various authors (1987) Artificial breeding in sheep and goats. *Proc. Univ. Sydney Post Grad Comm Vet. Sci.*, **96**

Laparoscopy

Van Reven, G. (1988) Laparoscopy in goats. *Goat Vet. Soc. J.*, **9** (1/2), 24–32

2 Abortion

Infectious causes of abortion

- Enzootic abortion (chlamydia).
- Toxoplasmosis.
- Listeriosis.
- Campylobacter (vibriosis).
- Q-fever.
- Leptospirosis.
- Salmonellosis.
- Tickborne fever.
- Border disease.
- Brucellosis.
- Sarcocystosis.

Non-infectious causes of abortion

- Medication.
- Trauma/stress.
- Developmental abnormalities.
- Multiple fetuses.
- Poisoning.
- Malnutrition.

Initial advice to owners

- Instruct the owner to save all the products of abortion for further examination – fetus/fetuses, fetal membranes. *The diagnosis will probably depend on laboratory investigation of aborted material.*
- Advise isolation of the aborted doe until a diagnosis is reached and/or uterine discharges have ceased.
- Warn of possible zoonoses, particularly during pregnancy. Care should be taken when handling aborted products – wear gloves. Any aborted material not required for laboratory examination should be burned or buried. Dogs and cats should be kept away from the aborted material.

Initial assessment

The preliminary history should consider:

- Individual or flock/herd problem.
- Possible exposure to infected animals – bought in stock etc.

Table 2.1 Causes of abortion

Abortion
Luteolysis
  trauma
  stress
Iatrogenic
  prostaglandins
  corticosteroids
Poisoning
Plant
Wormers
Infection
  enzootic abortion
  toxoplasmosis
  listeriosis
  campylobacter
  Q-fever
  leptospirosis
  salmonellosis
  tickborne fever
  border disease
  brucellosis
  sarcocystosis
Unknown
Nutrition
  starvation
  vitamin A deficiency
  manganese deficiency
Fetal developmental
abnormalities

- Feeding, e.g. silage.
- Vaccination.
- Known disease status.

Specific enquiries should cover.

- The length of gestation/timing of abortion (see Table 2.2).
- The general breeding history – return to service etc.
- The incidence of abortion, still births, weak kids.
- Signs of illness in the aborted doe.
- Drugs used on herd – e.g. prostaglandins.
- Access to possible poisons.
- The possibility of stress on the doe.

Table 2.2 Timing of abortion

Abortion throughout gestation

Toxoplasmosis
Chlamydia
Leptospirosis
Prostaglandins
Stress
Tickborne fever

Abortion in late gestation

Listeriosis
Campylobacter
Q-fever
Salmonellosis
Border disease
Corticosteroids
Multiple fetuses
Energy deficit
Mineral deficiency

Clinical examination

- The doe should be fully examined for signs of disease. Aborting does may be ill and the clinical signs may aid diagnosis, but because abortion may occur some time after infection, many aborting does will show few additional clinical signs. Abortion may follow acute septicaemia and pyrexia caused by conditions not normally associated with abortion, e.g. enterotoxaemia. A blood sample should be taken for laboratory investigation.
- The aborted fetuses and placentae should be examined grossly before submitting to the laboratory. If a number of does have aborted, samples from several animals should be submitted because of the possibility of more than one infectious agent being involved.

Laboratory investigation

Submission of correct specimens is essential for accurate diagnosis.

- Gross appearance of placentae and fetuses.

Submit:

(1) Placenta including colyledons – fresh or fixed in formol-saline
(2) Fresh fetuses or
   (a) fetal lung and liver – fresh and fixed
   (b) fetal abomasal contents – fresh
   (c) fetal heart blood or exudate from serous cavities – fresh
   (d) fetal brain – fixed.
- Demonstration of a pathogen, e.g. microscopy, direct culture, virus isolation.
- Serological examination of the dam.
- Serological examination of the fetus.

Infectious causes of abortion

- There are important differences between sheep and goats in the behaviour of some infectious organisms which cause abortion. Because the epidemiology of these conditions is different in the two species, the control measures taken to limit spread of disease in sheep will not necessarily be appropriate to goats.
- More than one infective agent may be involved in an abortion storm.

Enzootic abortion (chlamydia)

- Abortion occurs at any stage of pregnancy (unlike sheep where abortion is restricted to the last 2–4 weeks) because of the luteolytic effect from endometrial inflammation.
- The incubation period is as short as 2 weeks, so infection and abortion may occur within one pregnancy, even if infection occurs late in pregnancy.

Aetiology

- *Chlamydia psittaci,* an intracellular parasite of the Rickettsia family.

Transmission

- Ingestion of the organism shed in faeces but more generally from aborted material as Chlamydia is not very resistant in the environment.

- Carrier does or males in endemic herds and bought in does continue the spread of infection. Kids born live will also carry the infection, although they remain negative serologically, and may shed organisms when they kid themselves.

Clinical signs

Often abortion is the only clinical sign and the doe rapidly recovers but severe illness with metritis, keratoconjunctivitis and pneumonia has been reported.

Postmortem findings

- Placenta – intercotyledonary placentitis often with a covering of yellow purulent material, giving a leathery appearance. Advanced autolysis occurs.
- Fetus – no specific gross lesions occur; the fetus may be autolysed or fresh.

Laboratory diagnosis

- Examination of smears from the placenta, the mouth or nostrils of the fetus or the vagina of the doe using modified Ziehl Neelsen stain.
- Serological diagnosis of the disease using the complement fixation test, but males and young infected kids remain negative.
- Isolation of the organism in tissue culture or in embryonic eggs.

Treatment and control

- Segregate aborting animals for 2 weeks until the excretion of chlamydia has ceased.
- Dispose of aborted material and disinfect the area.
- Cull any live kids born to infected does.
- Treat all pregnant goats in the herd with tetracyclines for 10 days and move them to uncontaminated pasture halfway through the treatment.
- Consider a vaccination programme (ovine enzootic abortion vaccine, Coopers, Pitman-Moore). Vaccination of healthy females should prevent infection but may not prevent abortion in goats already infected.

Public health considerations

The organism is excreted in body fluids including milk. Pregnant women are particularly at risk from contact with aborted material and from drinking unpasteurized milk.

Toxoplasmosis

Aetiology

- *Toxoplasma gondii*, a protozoan parasite of endothelial cells.

Transmission

- Direct contact with the products of abortion.
- Infective oocysts passed in the faeces of cats which act as the intermediate host multiplying and disseminating infection and contaminating stored foodstuffs or pastures.

  A reservoir of infection for susceptible cats exists in birds and wild rodents, which may pass the infection vertically between generations. Cats then amplify and spread the infection.

- Transplacental infection of kids. Very low levels of infection may result in abortion.

Clinical signs

- Pyrexia and lethargy may occur in the doe about 2 weeks after infection, but the doe will be clinically normal at the time of abortion. Occasional fatalities occur in adult goats – postmortem findings include nephritis, cystitis, encephalitis, hepatitis, enteritis and abomasitis.
- Resorption, fetal death and mummification occur if infection is during the first third of pregnancy.
- Abortions, still births and weak kids are produced if infection occurs later in pregnancy.
- Normal but infected kids may be produced to does affected in late pregnancy.
- Up to 80% of females may be infected and abort.

Postmortem findings

- Placenta – yellow or white focal lesions 1–3 mm in diameter on the cotyledons with the intercotyledonary areas not affected.
- Fetus – there are usually no specific gross lesions on the fetus.

Laboratory diagnosis

- Fluorescent antibody examination of cotyledonary material.
- Examination of fetal fluid using latex agglutination test (available for practice laboratory use).
- Serological examination of dam may be confusing due to high serological levels in the normal population but rising titre between paired samples is indicative of infection and a low titre means that the abortion was not due to *Toxoplasma*.
- Serological examination of live kids before suckling will demonstrate high specific antibodies.
- Histological examination of fetal tissues – brain, lung, liver, heart, kidney and spleen – shows necrotic foci surrounded by inflammatory cells and focal leucomalocia in the brain.

Treatment and control

- Animals remain infected for life.
- Unlike sheep, infected goats may abort in subsequent pregnancies, so it may be advisable to cull infected does.
- Chemoprophylaxis with drugs such as monensin is likely to be of limited value in goats because of the risk of abortion during subsequent pregnancies (in sheep, 10–20 mg monensin per head per day may be included in the concentrate ration of pregnant ewes considered to be at risk).
- Infection can be prevented by stopping the access of cats to grain stores, feeding troughs and hay barns.
- Destroy the products of abortion as soon as possible.
- Oocysts may persist on pasture or in soil for over a year and are very resistant to most disinfectants.
- Cats acquire immunity to reinfection and do not subsequently present a threat to livestock unless they become immunosuppressed. Preventing cats breeding on the premises will prevent the spread of the disease via the intermediate host – younger cats generally pose the greatest threat.
- Rodent and bird control will reduce the reservoir of infection which exists for susceptible cats.

Public health considerations

Toxoplasma tachyzoites are passed in the milk of infected does, so there is a risk to children and pregnant women from drinking infected milk as well as from handling aborted material. Aborted material should never be handled with bare hands.

Listeriosis

See Chapter 11.

- Abortion occurs from the 12th week but generally in late pregnancy.
- Retained placentae and metritis are common after abortion.
- Some kids are born alive but die soon afterwards.

Postmortem findings

- Placenta – placentitis with cotyledons and intercotyledonary areas affected.
- Fetus – necrotic grey yellow foci 1–2 mm diameter in the liver and sometimes the lung.

Laboratory diagnosis

- The organism is easily grown and identified in the laboratory as a gram positive beta-haemolytic bacillus and can be isolated from the fetal stomach, uterine discharges, milk and the placenta.
- Fluorescent antibody examination of aborted material.

Treatment and control

- Clinically ill animals can be treated with ampicillin or trimethoprine sulphonamides
- Aborted does are considered immune and should be retained in the herd.

Campylobacter (Vibriosis)

Aetiology

- Comma shaped bacteria Campylobacter fetus (formerly Vibrio fetus). Campylobacter jejuni also implicated in USA.

Transmission

- Ingestion of organisms from aborted material.
- Some does remain permanent carriers.
- Wildlife can act as vectors.

Clinical signs

- Abortion in last 4–6 weeks of gestation; some infected goats do not abort but produce weak kids at full term. These kids usually die within a few days.

- Does may be pyrexic and lethargic with diarrhoea for a few days either side of the abortion, but often the goat appears clinically normal.
- A post abortion vaginal discharge is usual.
- Males are infected but do not show clinical signs.

Postmortem findings

- Placenta – changes minimal.
- Fetus – may have doughnut-shaped foci of 10–20 mm diameter in the liver; the fetus is usually autolysed.

Laboratory diagnosis

- Direct smear of fetal abomasal contents.
- Culture of fetal abomasal contents.

Treatment and control

- Segregate aborting animals immediately and then cull them because of the possibility of a carrier state.
- Cull any live kids born.
- Treat the remainder of the herd with penicillin/ dihydrostreptomycin or tetracyclines.

Public health consideration

- Campylobacter causes acute gastroenteritis in humans, usually by faecal contamination from diarrhoeic or apparently healthy goats. Faecal contamination of raw goats milk produced human disease in an outbreak in the UK.

Q-fever

Aetiology

- Very small intracellular parasite *Coxiella burnettii*, a member of the Rickettsia family.

Transmission

- By ingestion after direct contamination with abortion material or the urine, faeces and milk of an infected animal.
- By inhalation or through injured skin after contact with the organism.
- By infected ticks (?? UK).
- Healthy carrier goats spread the infection.

Clinical signs

- Most infected goats are healthy carriers but some aborting animals will be clinically ill with a retained placenta.
- Abortion occurs in the last month of pregnancy and weak infected kids may be born.

Postmortem findings

- Placenta – placentitis with clay coloured cotyledons and intercotyledonary thickening.
- Fetus – autolysed with no specific lesions.

Laboratory diagnosis

- Smears from the placenta or fetal organs stained with a modified Ziehl-Nielson stain show acid fast pleomorphic cocci and rods.
- By fluorescent antibody examination of cotyledonary material.
- A complement fixation test on the dam's serum shows the antibody level rising about a week after infections and persisting for a month.

Treatment and control

- Tetracyclines will probably control an outbreak.

Public health consideration

- The disease is most important as a human infection which occurs via contact or inhalation of the organism from the fetus, placenta and uterine fluids and possibly by drinking infected milk.

Leptospirosis

See Chapter 17.

Salmonellosis

Three Salmonella serotypes have been reported to cause abortion in sheep and goats – *S.abortus ovis, S.typhimurium, S.dublin*. The latter two cause systemic illness with diarrhoea in addition to abortion, still births or very weak live kids which die shortly afterwards.

Tickborne fever

Aetiology

- *Cytoecetes phagocytophilia*, an intracellular parasite of the Rickettsia family, transmitted by the tick vector *Ixodes ricinus*.

Epidemiology

- In endemic areas most ticks are infected and thus virtually all ruminants and deer exposed to ticks also become infected, generally very early in life.

Clinical signs

- Pyrexia, lethargy, weight loss (often not recognized).
- Abortion and metritis.
- Temporary infertility in male goats.

In addition, infection may increase the pathogenicity of other diseases such as tick pyaemia, louping ill, listeriosis, pasteurellosis etc.

- Anglo Nubian goats react more severely than other breeds of British goats.

Diagnosis

- Detection of the organism in polymorphonuclear leucocytes in Giemsa stained blood smears.

Control

- Susceptible pregnant animals should not be exposed to tick affected pastures.

Border disease (hypomyelinogenesis congenita, hairy shaker-disease)

Aetiology

- Pestivirus, serologically related to bovine virus diarrhoea and swine fever virus.

Epidemiology

- The incidence of the disease in the goat population is not known, but experimentally goats have been affected as well as sheep, and the virus should be considered as a possible cause of abortion. Direct animal contact by ingestion or aerosol is the main source of infection – sheep, goats, deer and possibly pigs are potential sources of infection. Surviving infected kids will remain carriers.

Clinical signs

- Abortion, still births, barren does, fetal death and maceration from 70th day.
- Small weak kids with varying degrees of tremor and abnormal conformation, although hairy coat abnormalities as seen in lambs rarely, if ever, occur.

Postmortem findings

- Kids – affected kids show hydrocephalus and cerebellar hypoplasia.
- Placenta – severe necrotizing caruncular placentitis.

Laboratory diagnosis

- Live animal: virus isolation and serology from kid or doe blood (clotted or heparinized).
- Postmortem: antigen can be detected in fresh samples of thyroid, kidney, brain, spleen, intestine, lymph nodes or placenta.
  virus can be isolated from postmortem material sent in virus transport medium.
  heart blood can be used for serology.
  histopathology of brain and spinal cord shows hypomyelinogenesis.

Brucellosis

Brucella abortus

Goats can be infected with *B.abortus* and hence are included in dairy cow testing programmes, but the incidence of infection is minute in all parts of the world. In infected goats abortion is rare and mastitis common. Serological testing of goats for brucellosis is reported to have severe limitations.

Brucella melitensis

Goats are most susceptible to *B.melitensis* which occurs mainly in Southern Europe and is important as a major zoonosis producing Malta fever in humans who drink infected milk.

Abortion is the main clinical sign and usually occurs during the last months of gestation. The organism is excreted in uterine and vaginal secretions, urine, faeces and milk after parturition or abortion.

Sarcocystosis

Aetiology

- *Sarcocystis capracanis*, a protozoan parasite using the goat as intermediate with a carnivore as definitive host.
  The incidence of the organism in the UK is unknown.

Clinical signs

- Depend on the number of sporocysts ingested.
- Clinical signs are non-specific and include pyrexia, anorexia, lethargy, haemolytic anaemia, jaundice, nervous signs and abortion due to maternal failure – placenta and fetus are not infected; weak kids may be born alive.

Diagnosis

- No antemortem diagnostic test is available.

Postmortem

- Non-specific findings; petechial haemorrhages in many organs.
- Haemorrhages in heart and skeletal muscle.
- Immunoflourescent and immunoperoxidase techniques used to identify PAS negative meronts in endothelial cells including the maternal carcuncle.

Other organisms which have been implicated in abortion are:

- *Corynebacterium pyogenes*
- *Yersinia pseudotuberculosis*
- *Pasteurella haemolytica*
- *Bacillus* spp.
- *Mycoplasma* spp.
- Caprine herpes virus

Non-infectious causes of abortion

Medication

- Prostaglandin administration will produce abortion at any stage of the gestation.

- Corticosteroids given in late pregnancy will also cause abortion.
- Phenothiazine used as a worm drench is reported to cause abortion in late pregnancy.

Trauma and stress

Goats may be more susceptible than other species to abortion from trauma or stress due to their dependence on the corpus luteum to maintain pregnancy. Any condition which causes release of prostaglandins, and thus luteolysis will cause abortion.

Developmental abnormalities

Very few deformed fetuses are produced but a fetus with developmental abnormalities may be aborted. An hereditary defect of Angora does in South Africa led to chronic hyperadrenocorticism, death of the fetus and then its expulsion.

Multiple fetuses

Abortions or early parturition appear more common in Anglo-Nubian goats which commonly carry 3, 4 or more fetuses. In these cases placental insufficiency probably leads to fetal expulsion.

Poisons

Plant poisonings are occasionally implicated in abortion, e.g. *Astragulus* spp. and *Lathyrus* spp., but are unlikely to be of significance in the UK. Poisonings from non-plant sources also occasionally occur, generally causing abortion by producing a systemic illness.

Nutrition

- *Energy deficit* – frank starvation will cause abortion particularly if the energy input is insufficient during the last third of pregnancy.
- *Mineral deficiencies* – mineral deficiencies, e.g. selenium, copper and iodine generally cause the birth of dead or weak kids at full term, rather than abortion but manganese deficiency has been shown to cause abortion at 80–105 days of gestation.

- *Vitamin deficiencies* – prolonged vitamin A deficiency has been shown to cause abortion, still birth, illthrift, retained placenta and night blindness due to the absence of visual purple in the retina. However deficiency is extremely unlikely even in severe drought.

Further reading

Abortion (general)

East, N. (1983) Pregnancy toxaemia, abortions and periparturent diseases. *Vet. Clin. North. Amer.: Large Anim. Pract.*, **5** (3), November 1983, Sheep and Goat Medicine, 601–618

Harwood, D. G. (1987) Abortion in the goat, an investigative approach. *Goat Vet. Soc. J.*, **8** (1), 25–28

Merrall, M. (1985) The aborting goat. *Proc. of a Course in Goat Husbandry and Medicine*. Massey University, November 1985, Publ. no. 106, 181–198

Campylobacter

Anderson, K. L., Hammond, M. M., Urbane, J. W., Rhoades, H. E. and Bryner, J. H. (1983) Isolation of *Campylobacter jejuni* from an aborted caprine fetus. *JAVMA*, **183**, 90–92

Chlamydial abortion

Appleyard, W. T. (1986) Chlamydial abortion in goats. *Goat Vet. Soc. J.*, **7** (2), 45–47

Q-fever

Waldhalm, D. G., Stoenner, H. G., Simmons, E. E. and Thomas, A. L. (1978) Abortion associated with *Coxiella burnettii* infection in dairy goats. *JAVMA*, **173**, 1580–1581

Toxoplasmosis

Buxton, D. (1989) Toxoplasmosis in sheep and other farm animals. *In Practice*, January 1989, 9–12

Dubey, J. P., Miller, S. and Desmonts, G. (1986) *Toxoplasma gondii* induced abortion in dairy goats. *JAVMA*, **188**, 159–162

Herbert, I. V. (1986) Sarcocystosis and toxoplasmosis in goats. *Goat Vet. Soc. J.*, **7** (2), 25–31

3 Male infertility

Initial assessment
Individual buck problems

Initial assessment

The preliminary history should consider:

- Individual or flock/herd problem.
- Management practices – handmating/buck running with does.
- Feeding, including mineral supplementation.
- Workload of the bucks.
- Age of bucks.

If more than one buck is involved consider:

- Overuse of bucks – particularly if used out of season or on synchronized groups of does. One buck can mate over 100 does over a season, but a ratio of one mature buck to about 70 does or two bucklings (two toothbucks) to 70 does is more satisfactory. A well grown kid could serve up to 30 does in a season.
- Low sexual drive – if bucks used out of season on light treated or sponged does.
- Disease status – parasitism, footrot etc.
- Nutritional status.
- Poor heat detection.

If there is a problem with an individual goat, the specific history should determine whether the problem is:

- Return to service of females.
- Failure to serve at all.
- Failure to serve properly.

Examination of the buck

- Observe sexual activity using doe in season as teaser (prostaglandin treatment of doe during breeding season can be used to induce oestrus at a time suitable for examination).
      libido
      failure to mate
- General clinical examination
      body condition
      arthritis
      weak pasterns
      poorly trimmed feet

- Examination and palpation of external genitalia
  check the scrotum and contents; note the size, shape, consistency and symmetry of the testes, epididymis and spermatic cord; the testes should move freely in the scrotum.
  measure the scrotal circumference and the epididymal diameter.

Table 3.1 Causes of male infertility

Male infertility
History
Herd/flock problem
  overuse of bucks
  out of season breeding
  disease
  nutrition
  poor heat detection
Individual buck problem
Failure to serve
  low libido
  failure to mount
    laminitis
    footrot
    overgrown feet
    arthritis
    weak pasterns
    back pain
Failure to serve properly
  failure to gain intromission
    balanoposthitis
    phimosis
    persistent frenulum
    penile haematoma
    short penis
  failure to thrust
    stress
    overweight
    back pain
Return to service
of females
  poor sperm quality
    overuse
    age
    nutrition
    disease
    abnormal testicles
    abnormal epididymis
    abnormal accessory
      sex glands

Scrotum

Scrotal dermatitis, abscesses, fly strike and trauma can all lead to temporary or permanent testicular degeneration and reduced fertility.

Testes

The testes should be symmetrical, large, oval and firm during the breeding season. Asymmetry suggests injury, disease or anatomical abnormality.

Cryptorchidism

Cryptorchidism may be unilateral or bilateral. Unilateral cryptorchids are generally fertile but semen quality may be affected; bilateral cryptorchids are sterile. A genetically female intersex may be a cryptorchid. In Angora goats cryptorchidism has been shown to be inherited as a recessive trait.

Enlarged testes

- An inguinal hernia causing distension of the scrotum may be confused with enlarged testicles.
- *Orchitis* – inflammation of the testes may be unilateral or bilateral, acute or chronic. In the acute condition, the testes will be swollen and painful and the buck will be pyrexic, lethargic and unwilling to move. In chronic orchitis, fibrous adhesions may limit movement within the scrotum and the testicles become atrophied and fibrous.
- *Neoplasia* – an uncommon cause of infertility in bucks but seminomas, adenomas and carcinomas have been reported.
- *Haematoma* – intratesticular haemorrhage may cause enlargement of a testis.

Small testes

- *Testicular hypoplasia* – underdeveloped testes occur particularly in polled males as part of the intersex condition (qv). The condition is generally bilateral, occasionally unilateral.
- *Testicular atrophy* – occurs as a sequel to scrotal trauma, orchitis, sperm granuloma or systemic disease, if the goat is debilitated and as part of the ageing process in some bucks. With fibrosis the testicle feels very firm on palpation.
- *Testicular degeneration* – the testes feel soft and doughy due to tubular degeneration.

Conditions of spermatic cord

- *Varicocoele* – presents as a hard swelling in dorsal part of the pampiniform plexus; caused by dilation and thrombosis in the internal spermatic vein.

Abnormal epididymis

- *Sperm granulomas* are palpable as hard knots at the head of the epididymis although the testes are normal in consistency. The condition occurs particularly in polled males as part of the intersex condition (qv) but can also arise from an infection causing epididymitis. If the condition is bilateral the buck is sterile.
- *Epididymitis* uncommonly occurs in goats as a result of infection with a variety of pathogens or following trauma.

Penis/prepuce

Balanoposthitis

- Inflammation of the penis and prepuce often leads to scar tissue and adhesions. The acute inflammation and the resulting fibrosis both cause infertility.
- *Caprine herpes virus type 1* causes balanoposthitis in goats in New Zealand and Australia with hyperaemia of the penis and ulceration of the prepuce.
- *Orf* (qv) occasionally infects the prepuce.
- Mycoplasmas and ureaplasms *may* be involved.

Persistent frenulum

The adhesions between the penis and prepuce which are present in the prepubertal male kid, normally disappear by about 4 months of age, but occasionally persist.

Phimosis

Phimosis is seen as an inability to extrude the penis at service. It may result from trauma but is occasionaly congenital.

Paraphimosis

Paraphimosis is the inability to withdraw the penis into the prepuce, resulting in the penis becoming swollen and oedematous.

Short penis

This results in inability to protrude the penis beyond the prepuce. The condition is not treatable.

Haematoma of penis

This follows trauma such as headbutting.

Examination of semen

- Collection of semen
    using an artificial vagina gives better quality semen than electroejaculation; if possible use doe in oestrus as teaser.
    electroejaculation should only be used on an anaesthetized animal.
    best semen samples are obtained during the breeding season.
    some idea of sperm motility can be gained from a vaginal semen sample examined on a warmed slide.
- Examination of semen – volume, motility, numbers, morphology, absence of inflammatory cells/debris, live:dead ratio (see Appendix, 7)

Individual buck problems

Failure to serve at all

Low libido

- Season – the normal breeding season is September to March, but many bucks are now expected to work out of season following light or sponge treatment of does. If possible bucks should be stimulated, e.g. by light, at the same time as the does. Most bucks will mate at any time of the year, but some reduction in libido must be expected out of season.
- Poor condition – intercurrent disease such as parasitizm; energy or protein deficit.
- Hereditary – sexual drive is heritable.
- Presence of other males. Competition may increase libido, or a dominant male may suppress libido in subordinates.

Note: many (particularly older) bucks will only serve a female that is defintely in season. Some bucks will only serve each female once within a short period of time rather than twice as expected by dairy goat keepers.

Failure to mount

- Skeletal or muscular lesions:
  foot problems: laminitis, footrot, overgrown feet
  arthritis
  back pain
  weak pasterns.

Failure to serve properly

Failure to gain intromission

- Conditions of prepuce – phimosis due to trauma or infection, persistent frenulum (rare), adhesions/scarring.

Note A very young male kid (<4 months) may have difficulty protruding the penis because of adhesions between penis and prepuce.

- Conditions of penis – adhesions/scarring, haematoma, short penis.

Failure to thrust

- Stress – too many people 'assisting'
  tiredness
  strange surroundings.
- Overweight.
- Back pain.

Return to service

Generally caused by poor sperm quality.

- Overuse – particularly out of season and if large numbers of does synchronized; reduced sperm density may take 6 weeks or more to recover.
- Age – old or young animal may have reduced sperm density, and/or poor quality semen.
- Start of breeding season – maximum sperm production occurs several weeks after onset of season.
- Nutrition – young males are particularly sensitive to poor nutrition including protein and energy deficits and vitamin deficiency (particularly Vitamin A). The role of trace elements is not well documented but copper, manganese, cobalt, zinc and phosphorus deficiences may affect sperm production.
- Stress.

- Intercurrrent disease – pyrexia will reduce sperm density through damage to epididymis and testes causing permanent damage in some cases and a minimum of 6 weeks to recover. The spermatogenic cycle is about 22 days in the goat and normal fertility is not restored until a full spermatogenic cycle is completed.
- Abnormal testicles.
- Abnormal epididymis.
- Abnormal accessory sex glands, e.g. *seminal vesiculitis* – results in ejaculates containing large numbers of white cells with no palpable orchitis or epididymitis.
- Heavy fibre cover – an unshorn Angora with heavy fleece may have reduced fertility due to increase in scrotal temperature and affect on spermatogenesis. Even after shearing 6–8 weeks will be required before return to full fertility.

Further reading

General

Evans, G. and Maxwell, W. M. C. (1987) *Salamon's Artificial Insemination of Sheep and Goats*. Butterworths, London

Greig, A. (1987) Infertility in the male goat. *Goat Vet. Soc. J.*, **8** (1), 1–3

Merman, M. A. (1983) Male infertility. *Vet. Clin. North Amer.: Large Animal Practice*, **5** (3), November 1983, 619–635

4 Periparturient problems

Preparturient problems

Pregnancy toxaemia
Dead kids without immediate abortion
Abortion
Vaginal prolapse
Rectal prolapse
Prolonged gestation
Dystocia
Hypocalcaemia
Hypomagnesaemia
Transit tetany

Postparturient problems

Metritis
Retained placenta
Retained kid
Rupture of the uterus
Ruptured uterine artery
Uterine prolapse
Hypocalcaemia
Mastitis
Postparturient toxaemia
Laminitis

Preparturient problems

Pregnancy toxaemia

See Chapter 8.

Dead kids without immediate abortion

Retention of a dead or mummified kid is not uncommon in goats. Kids may be retained for several months before the doe produces a macerated kid or bones. Small pieces of bone may be retained in the uterus and cause infertility. Occasionally mummified kids are found incidentally at postmortem.

Retention of a non-mummifed kid will produce an acute toxaemia with pyrexia, anorexia, abdominal pain and usually death within about 3 days. Intermittent straining may occur terminally. If the cervix is closed internal examination is not possible, radiography will confirm the diagnosis.

Abortion

See Chapter 2.

Vaginal prolapse

This is relatively common. Likely to recur during subsequent pregnancies with probable increasing severity, but some goats prolapse only once. Generally kid normally without subsequent prolapse of the uterus.

Aetiology

• An increase in intrapelvic pressure in late pregnancy initiates straining by the doe, forcing vagina through the vulva. Factors implicated in increasing the likelihood of prolapse include:

  multiple fetuses
  conformation of dam – musculature,
  pelvic anatomy, ? hereditary component
    in goats, overfatness is generally not significant.

Clinical signs

• Degree of prolapse is variable from a minor protrusion of the vagina through the vulval lips when lying down to a complete prolapse of the vagina and cervix in which the bladder may also be prolapsed.

Treatment

• Minor prolapses – no treatment provided the area remains untraumatized and clean.
• Larger prolapse – suture vulval lips with nylon tape after cleaning and reduction of the prolapse.
• Complete prolapse – reduce under epidural anaesthesia, suture vulva or in Angora goats use metal or plastic ewe womb retainer tied to fleece.
• Consider early induced parturition with prostaglandins (qv) if the goat is distressed.

- Sutures should be cut when kidding commences – needs regular checks once pelvic ligaments relax; consider induction of parturition for fairly accurate timing of the delivery.

Note: *Prolapse of the intestines through a vaginal rupture* may occur if a portion of the intestines is forced into the pelvis.

Rectal prolapse

Rare; may follow vaginal prolapse if straining occurs.

Prolonged gestation

The normal gestation period is 150 days (145–154 days).

Single kids are often carried longer than multiples. If parturition has not occurred by 155 days, parturition should be induced with prostaglandins (qv) and will result in kidding in about 36 hours. Hypocalcaemia (qv) should always be considered and treated where necessary.

Common causes of prolonged gestation are:

- Non-pregnancy!
- Hydrometra (qv).
- Single large kid.
- Dead kids.
- Hypocalcaemia.

Dystocia

Generally due to malpresentation (particularly with multiple fetuses), occasionally to an oversize fetus or to overfat does, particularly goatlings.

True 'ringwomb' where the cervix fails to dilate sufficiently to allow parturition is rare but manual dilation of the vulva, vagina and cervix may be necessary where the fetus has not engaged correctly in the pelvis, e.g. with a transverse presentation. In some cases 3 ml Monzaldon (Boehringer Ingelheim) will aid dilation. Hypocalcaemia should always be considered.

The uterus of the goat is more readily damaged than that of the ewe. Adequate lubrication and dilatation of the canal is essential or rupture of the cervix with dorsal tearing of the uterus and possibly uterine haemorrhage will occur. If in doubt a caesarian section is indicated!

Hypocalcaemia
See Chapter 11.

Hypomagnesaemia
See Chapter 11.

Transit tetany
See Chapter 11.

Postparturient problems
Metritis
- A light odourless reddish discharge (lochia) is *normal* for about 14 days after parturition and does not indicate metritis. Metritis is indicated by a darker, sticky usually smelly discharge which may contain pus. The doe may be pyrexic andanorexic with a reduced milk yield and signs of abdominal pain.
- Does which progress to chronic metritis may be infertile (see Chapter 1).

Retained placenta
- Much less common than in the cow; induction of parturition with prostaglandins does not lead to retention.
- Fetal membranes should be passed within 12 hours. After this time immediate veterinary intervention is necessary as contraction of the uterus and closure of the cervix will soon prevent manual removal. Injections of oxytocin or prostaglandin may aid removal of the membranes. Antibiotic cover should be given routinely and tetanus antitoxin given in unvaccinated goats.

Retained kid
See Preparturient problems.

Rupture of the uterus
- Usually occurs dorsally in the body of the uterus just cranial to the cervix.

- Repair of a dorsal tear is extremely difficult either by a left flank abdominal incision or vaginally. However, in many cases, contraction of the uterus will seal the defect and the doe may not only survive but breed and kid satisfactorily in subsequent years. The main dangers are shock and peritonitis – the fetal membranes should be removed as completely as possible,high levels of intravenous antibiotics given and pain relief given as isopyrin/phenylbutazone (Tomanol, Intervet) 3–5 ml i.v. or flunixin meglumine (Finadyne, Schering Plough) 2 ml/45 kg i.v. or aspirin 50–100 mg/kg orally t.i.d.

Ruptured uterine artery

- Rare; may accompany a ventral tear of the uterus or occur during a difficult kidding. Fatal intraperitoneal haemorrhage can occur without obvious vaginal haemorrhage.

Uterine prolapse

- Rare: occurs a few hours after kidding often subsequent to a retained placenta.
- If the placenta is still attached, it should be gently removed before thorough cleaning and replacement under epidural anaesthesia. The horns of the uterus must be fully extended when replaced.
- The vulval lips can be sutured together, or a purse string suture used or a ewe womb retainer inserted.

Hypocalcaemia

See Chapter 11.

Mastitis

See Chapter 12.

Postparturient toxaemia

See Chapter 8.

Laminitis

See Chapter 6.

Further reading

Baxendell, S. A. (1984) Caprine obstetrics. *Proc. Univ. Sydney. Post Grad Comm. Vet. Sci.*, **73**, 363–366

Brain, L. T. A. (1985) Dystocia in the goat – a practitioner's view. *Goat Vet. Soc. J.*, **6** (2), 57–60

East, N. E. (1983) Pregnancy toxaemia, abortions and periparturient diseases. *Vet. Clin. North Amer.: Large Animal Practice*, **5** (3), November 1983, 601–618

Noakes, D. E. (1985) Surgical answers to reproductive problems in the female goat. *Goat Vet. Soc. J.*, **6** (2), 61–63

5 Weak kids

Initial assessment
Clinical examination
Prematurity/low birth weight
Birth injury
Malnutrition
Congenital defects
Infection
Exposure

Weak kids result from a number of causes, many of which may be interrelated. Thus a kid which is premature or has a developmental abnormality may have difficulty suckling and succumb to starvation and secondary hypothermia.

- Prematurity.
- Low birth weight.
- Birth injury.
- Malnutrition.

    Intrauterine
        copper deficiency (enzootic ataxia)
        iodine deficiency (goitre)
        selenium deficiency (white muscle disease)

    Postnatal
        inability to suckle
        mismothering
        agalactia
        poor udder conformation
        teat abnormalities

- Congenital defects
    Genetic
        atresia ani
        arthrogryposis (contracted tendons)
        microphthalmia
        hydrocephalus
        cerebellar hypoplasia
        (mannosidosis)

    Development abnormalities
        hyper/hypoflexion of limbs
        ventricular septal defect
        hydronephrosis
        cleft palate
        spinal abnormalities

- Infection
    Congenital
        Chlamydia
        Salmonella
        Toxoplasmosis
        Listeriosis
        Q-fever
        Border disease
        Sarcocystis

Postnatal
- *Escherichia coli*
- Clostridia
- Pasteurella
- *Staphylococcus aureus*
- *Streptococcus* spp.
- *Corynebacterium* spp.
- Tick pyaemia

- Exposure
  - Primary hypothermia
  - Secondary hypothermia

Initial assessment

The preliminary history should consider:
- Individual or flock/herd problem.
- Kidding routine.
- Post kidding management.
- Beginning or end of kidding period.
- Feeding.

If a flock/herd problem consider:
- Associated abortions/still births.
- Possible nutritional deficiencies.

If an individual problem specific enquiries should cover:
- Weak since birth or developed since?
- Seen to suckle or not.
- Difficult or prolonged birth.
- Kidded inside or outside – possibility of exposure.

Clinical examination

Observe kid and dam together in their normal surroundings
- Mismothering – particularly first kidders.
- Behaviour of siblings.
- Sucking reflex.

Examine dam

- Udder conformation/teat abnormalities.
- Milk let down.
- Mastitis.
- Vaginal discharges.

Examine kid

- Alert?
- Check for congenital lesions.
- Nervous signs.

Prematurity/low birth weight

Birth weights of kids are very variable, ranging from over 7 kg for a single male down to 2.0 or 3.0 kg in multiple births. Birth weight is important as the larger the kid at birth the faster the growth rate.

Kids up to 14 days premature have a good chance of survival and kids up to 21 days premature can often be reared.

Premature kids may have respiratory problems due to inadequate lung surfactant being produced. This is particularly the case if parturition is induced with prostaglandins before about day 144 of gestation.

Birth injury

At birth the kid undergoes some quite profound changes to enable it to adapt to its new environment. With the exception of the development of the rumen the major physiological changes are over by a few days after birth and any associated signs of maladjustment appear by this time. It is quite possible that the kid will have to compensate for the deleterious effects of parturition itself.

- *Trauma* from the physical forces of parturition or from traction in an assisted birth.
- *Compression* of the kid's thorax as it passes through the pelvis causing compression of the lungs.
- *Asphyxia* from pressure on the umbilical cord during passage through the pelvic cavity or from reduced efficiency of the placenta during uterine contractions.

Birth injury can result directly in the death of a kid if the damage is severe enough, e.g. from abdominal haemorrhage due to liver rupture, or difficulty in breathing, or may lead to death from starvation/hypothermia by impairing feeding and movement.

Malnutrition

Intrauterine deficiencies

Copper deficiency (enzootic ataxia, swayback)

Aetiology

- Copper deficiency, either as a result of copper deficient soils or, generally in the UK as a result of a conditioned deficiency with reduced copper utilization by the grazing animals, e.g. pasture topdressing with molybdenum and sulphur which reduce the availability of copper, or heavy lime applications which increase pasture molybdenum intake and thus reduce the copper intake. It is a disease of grazing animals or animals fed grass-based diets and home-produced cereals. Zero grazed animals receiving a concentrate ration are unlikely to be affected.

  Although the clinical signs and pathological lesions are similar to those in lambs, in goat herds clinical cases tend to be sporadic rather than a flock problem as in sheep and there is less correlation between copper levels and clinical disease.

Clinical signs

(1) Congenital form
   - Kid is affected at birth. Some kids may be of low viability and succumb to hypothermia without showing marked neurological signs.
(2) Delayed form
   - Clinical signs do not appear until the kid is several weeks or even months old.
   - Bright, alert, willing to suck and eat.
   - Muscle tremors, head shaking.
   - Progressive hind limb ataxia, progressing to paralysis.
   - Adult goats in the same herd may have anaemia, diarrhoea, poor fleece quality and fail to thrive.

- Other kids may show growth retardation, increased susceptibility to infections, poor fleece quality and susceptibility to fractures (distinguish from parasitism, cobalt deficiency or inadequate nutrition).

Diagnosis

- Clinical signs.
- Plasma copper levels >9.0 µmol/l adequate.
- CSF within normal limits.
- Histological examination of the CNS.
- Liver copper levels (normal >40 mg/kg DM).

Low liver copper levels may occur in some kids without enzootic ataxia and some apparently affected kids appear to have normal levels (due to subsequent supplementation?).

Postmortem findings

- Generally no gross pathology of nervous system.
- Demyelination of cerebellar and spinal cord tracts.
- Cerebellar corticol hypoplasia; necrosis and loss of Purkinje cells of cerebellum.
- Chromatolytic necrosis in brain stem nuclei and spinal cord.
- May be skeletal abnormalities – brittle bones, healing rib fractures.

Treatment

- Often unsuccessful except early in the disease; may prevent further deterioration in delayed form.
- Copper administration
    - (i) injection – Copavet (C.Vet), Cujec (Coopers Pitman-Moore)
    - (ii) oral – Copacaps (RMB Animal Health), Copacobal oral drench (C.Vet).

Note: Overdosage with copper causes toxicity (qv) so supplementation should be used with care and manufacturers' recommendations followed.

Prevention

- Soil and plant analysis for copper and its antagonists molybdenum, sulphur and iron and correction by fertilizer applications under professional advice.

- Copper supplementation to does during early pregnancy:
    - (1) injections – Copavet (C.Vet), Cujec (Coopers Pitman-Moore), Cuvine (Rycovet)
    - (2) oral – Copacaps (RMB), Copacobal oral drench (C.Vet), Copporal (Smith Kline Beecham)
    - (3) water additives – Aquatrace Copper tablets (Denis Brinicombe).

Iodine deficiency (goitre)

Goitre is commonly misdiagnosed by goatkeepers when kids have any enlargement in the throat region (see chapter 9). In particular, thymic swellings, which are common, regularly lead to a misdiagnosis. True iodine deficiency is probably rare in the UK. Angoras are more susceptible than dairy goats or sheep.

Aetiology

- Natural deficiencies of iodine.
- Goitrogenic feeds, e.g. kale and cabbage produce a secondary iodine deficiency by accumulation of isothiocyanates which prevent the accumulation of iodine in the thyroid gland.

Clinical signs

- Abortion.
- Still births or very weak kids born at term or slightly early with thin sparse hair coat; susceptible to cold stress, respiratory problems.
- Enlarged thyroid glands (goitre) in the affected kids produce palpable swellings posterior and ventral to the larynx (more discrete than thymic glands involving distal rather than proximal cervical region). The thyroid may weigh between 10 and 50 g compared to the normal weight of 2 g.
- A subclinical deficiency may result in small weak kids without obvious goitre.
- Older goats in the herd may show decreased production, poor growth rate and reduced appetite.
- Iodine deficiency may also result in subfertility.

Diagnosis

- Blood thyroxine assay.

Prevention and treatment

- Iodized saltlicks or loose iodized salt in the diets of older goats will prevent development of iodine deficiency. Alternatively, dose with potassium iodide 2 months and 2 weeks before kidding – dissolve 20 g of potassium iodide in 1 litre of water and dose at a rate of 10 ml per 20 kg liveweight.
- Affected kids can be treated with 3–5 drops of Lugol's iodine in milk daily for one week.
- Avoid goitrogenic feeds such as kale.

Iodine toxicity: treatment of goats incorrectly diagnosed by the owner as being iodine deficient can lead to iodine toxicity which produces anorexia, lacrimation, coughing, dandruff in the coat and weight loss.

Selenium deficiency

Kids may occasionally have signs of white muscle disease (qv) at birth.

Postnatal malnutrition

Where the dam is failing to provide sufficient milk for whatever reason the kid should be removed, stomach tubed and bottle fed as necessary.

Congenital defects

Many congenital defects will be incompatible with satisfactory growth and development. An exception is hyper/hypoflexion of limbs (qv) which will often correct themselves within a few days although some will need splinting. Kids which cannot suckle their dam should be bottle fed.

β.*mannosidosis* is an inherited lysosomal disease attributable to an autosomal recessive gene which has been reported in Australia, New Zealand, USA, Fiji and Canada but not the UK. Because of the absence of the enzyme β.mannosidase, kids are unable to stand from birth due to carpal contractures and hyperextended fetlocks. Withdrawal reflexes are normal but movement is accompanied by an intention tremor. Kids may show domed skulls, narrow muzzles and palpebral fissures.

Infection

Congenital

Weak kids may be born as part of clinical syndromes involving abortions and still births. These infections include toxoplasmosis, Q-fever, chlamydiosis and Border disease. These are discussed under Chapter 2, Abortion.

Infections acquired after birth

In the first few hours after birth, the kid is susceptible to infection from a number of infective agents which gain access via the navel or mouth resulting in infection of the navel, septicaemia, pyaemia, enteritis and joint ill. Possible organisms involved include *Escherichia coli, Clostridium perfringens* type B, *Staphylococcus aureus, Streptococcus* spp., *Corynebacterium* spp., *Salmonella* and rotavirus.

Many other organisms are potential pathogens. Infection is more likely in intensive kidding systems, particularly towards the end of the kidding period.

Exposure

Primary hypothermia

Direct exposure of kids to cold, wet, windy weather so heat loss exceeds heat production. Small kids have a relatively large surface area relative to body weight and relatively small energy reserves and so are more prone to hypothermia than large kids.

Secondary hypothermia

Most kids who die from hypothermia succumb to secondary hypothermia where the neonates are unable to suckle and replenish their body reserves in weather which is insufficiently cold to kill through primary hypothermia. Thus mismothering, agalactia, birth injury etc can all lead to death from secondary hypothermia.

Hypoglycaemia can be reversed by an intraperitoneal injection of a 20% glucose solution at a rate of 10 ml/kg. Holding the kid by its front legs inject 1 cm to the side and 2 cm behind the umbilicus with the needle directed at a 45° angle towards the rump, using a 50 ml syringe and 19 g 2.5 cm needle.

NB   (1) Deeply hypothermic kids over 5 hours old are likely to be seriously hypoglycaemic. Treating the hypoglycaemia in these kids before warming is essential to prevent death from cerebral hypoglycaemia.

(2) Colostrum can be fed by stomach tube at a rate of 50-75 ml/kg, i.e. 150-250 ml per feed or until the stomach feels full on palpation.

Further reading

Anon (1982) Detection and treatment of hypothermia in newborn lambs. *In Practice*, January 1982, 20–22
Eales, A. (1987) Feeding lambs by stomach tube. *In Practice*, January 1987, 18–20
Matthews, J. G. (1985) Care of the newborn kid. *Goat Vet. Soc. J.*, **6** (2), 64–67
Papworth, S. M. (1981) The young kid. *Goat Vet. Soc. J.*, **2** (2), 12–15

6 Lameness in adult goats

Foot

Infectious diseases

- Interdigital dermatitis.
- Foot rot.
- Foot abscess.
- Orf.
- Mycotic dermatitis (strawberry footrot).
- Foot and mouth disease.

Non-infectious diseases

- White line disease.
- Bruising/trauma to hoof.
- Foreign body.
- Fractured pedal bone.
- Laminitis.

Above the foot

Weak pasterns

Accident or trauma

- Fracture.
- Soft tissue damage
  rupture of the superficial and deep digital flexor tendons
  rupture of the peroneus tertius muscle
  rupture of the cranial cruciate ligament
  luxating patella
  radial nerve injury

Lameness after injection

Carpal hygroma

Osteopetrosis

Degenerative arthritis (osteoarthritis)

Caprine arthritis encephalitis

Lameness

As in most other farm animals, the majority of cases of lameness in goats involve the foot and the majority of foot lameness in both dairy goats and fibre goats results from *poor foot care*. *Conformation problems* such as weak pasterns or cowhocks will predispose to uneven hoof growth and environmental factors such as excessively wet conditions which soften the horn, may lead to excessive horn growth and increase susceptibility to infection. However, the cornerstone of lameness prevention within a herd remains regular routine foot trimming. Tetanus is a possible sequel to any penetrating infection, particularly of the foot and adequate antitetanus cover should always be given.

Investigating the lame goat

Initial assessment

The preliminary history should consider:

- Individual or flock/herd problem.
- Sudden or gradual onset of lameness.
- Duration of lameness.
- Static or progressive lameness.
- Any predisposing factors such as excessively wet conditions.

Clinical examination

The animal should be examined at rest and while moving from a distance of a few feet for:

- Weight bearing.
- Stance.
- Obvious wounds, swellings etc.
- Conformation.
- Overgrown feet.

A detailed examination should then localize the seat of the lameness by:

- Cleaning and trimming the feet where necessary.
- Palpation.
- Manipulation.

Additional information can be obtained from radiography or laboratory examination as indicated.

Treatment

- Specific treatment should be instigated as soon as a diagnosis is made.

- Ensure feet are correctly trimmed.
- Instigate pain relief/anti-inflammatory treatment as indicated.
  (1) Flunixin meglumine (Finadyne, Schering Plough) –
      2 ml/45 kg i.v. or i.m. every 12 or 24 hours for up to 5 days.
  (2) Phenylbutazone – 4 mg/kg i.v. or p.o. every 12–24 hours.
  (3) Isopyrin/phenylbutazone (Tomanol, Intervet) 3–5 ml i.v.
  (4) Aspirin 50–100mg/kg p.o. t.i.d.

Infectious disease of the foot

Interdigital dermatitis/footrot

Predisposing conditions:

- Prolonged grazing of wet, muddy pastures, or housing in wet dirty yards.
- Overcrowding.
- Introduction of new stock – infection may be introduced by clinical or subclinical carriers (goats, sheep, cattle or deer).
- Poor foot care.
- Poor foot conformation.

Aetiology

- Continuous wetting of the foot and interdigital skin damages the tissues and allows the invasion of the causal organism of *interdigital dermatitis, Fusobacterium necrophorum. F. necrophorum* is widespread in the environment and cannot penetrate healthy intact skin. Its penetration is aided by other bacteria such as *Corynebacterium pyogenes*.
- Interdigital dermatitis may exist as a distinct condition but in the presence of *Bacteroides nodosus*, which is introduced by carrier animals, there is a rapid spread of the infection to the hoof and the sole and *benign footrot* or *virulent footrot* becomes established. *B. nodosus*, which acts synergistically with *F. necrophorum*, has a varying keratinolytic activity which destroys the hoof, permitting further invasion of the foot. When strains with low keratinolytic activity are present damage will be limited and only the mild lesions of benign footrot seen. When the strains have high keratinolytic activity, damage is much more severe and virulent footrot occurs.

Interdigital dermatitis (Scald)

Goats, with longer digits and a deeper interdigital area, show more severe clinical signs than sheep.

Clinical signs

- A mild to severe lameness in one or more goats with a rapid spread throughout the flock or herd if the predisposing conditions are suitable; animals will be lame in one or more feet, or walking on their knees. Affected animals will lose condition with drop in milk yield or shedding of fleece.
- The interdigital area between the claws is inflamed, often with considerable swelling, and there is a characteristic smell. There is no damage to the horn of the hoof. In severe cases there will be ulceration with a purulent discharge.

Footrot

Clinical signs

- As for interdigital dermatitis, but there are lesions in the hoof and sole, with separation of the horn, caused by underrunning. In severe cases the hoof will only be attached at the coronet. Pus is present beneath the underrun horn and the horn can be pared away revealing greyish soft horn with a characteristic foul odour of decomposing tissue.

  Secondary complications may arise from fly strike or tetanus.

Treatment and control

- Regular examination and foot trimming of the whole herd.
- Uncomplicated cases of interdigital dermatitis will resolve quickly if the animals are moved from wet pasture to dry ground or housed and the lesions treated with an antibiotic spray or footbath.
- If footrot is present the feet of infected goats should be trimmed separately and the footrot shears disinfected between goats. All infected and underrun tissue should be removed. Foot parings should be disposed of carefully.
- If an individual goat is affected dip the feet in a footbath solution daily for 3 days and then weekly for several weeks. Local antibiotic aerosol sprays, together with parenteral antibiotic therapy is sometimes useful and a severely affected foot can be bandaged. A zinc sulphate/vaseline mixture can be applied locally interdigitally.
- With a herd problem, the goats should be run through a footbath on a weekly basis. Goats need to be closely supervised as they are much more adept at avoiding the bath than sheep. The bath should be at least 4 cm deep and the

goats should stand in the bath for at least 2 minutes routinely and for 30 minutes when the infection is severe.

Three solutions are commonly used:

Copper sulphate 10% (Bluestone)	– 10 kg copper sulphate to 100 litres water.
Formalin 5–10%	– 5–10 litres commercial formalin (formalin 40%) to 100 litres water.
Zinc sulphate 10%	– 10 kg zinc sulphate to 100 litres water.

Formalin is very effective but stings raw tissue and makes the goats less amenable to adequate bathing and also hardens the skin and hoof, possibly preventing the penetration of further solutions. Copper sulphate may stain fleeces and may also cause toxicity in goats which drink from the footbath. Zinc sulphate solution is thus the preferred treatment, although a longer bathing period is required than with formalin and the solution is more expensive. Footrite (Veterinary Pharmaceuticals) is a zinc preparation containing a penetrating agent to increase the deposition of zinc in the hoof.

The goats should be penned on dry ground until their feet are dry.

- Parenteral chemotherapy – advisable in severe cases; use penicillin/streptomycin or tetracyclines.
- Vaccination – footrot vaccines (Clovax, Footvax, Coopers Pitman-Moore) have been used with very mixed results. Vaccination alone will *not* control the disease.

  Severe local reactions to the oil adjuvanted Footvax have been reported.
- Select for resistance. There is some evidence that there are family and breed differences in the incidence of footrot, possibly related to foot conformation.

Foot abscess

Predisposing conditions:

- Injury to the foot from stones, overzealous trimming, puncture wounds etc.
- The presence of interdigital dermatitis/footrot.
- White line disease.
- Sandcracks in the hoof wall (particularly lateral side of hoof).

Aetiology
- As a sequel to interdigital dermatitis/footrot or a penetration wound of the foot, deep infection by *C. pyogenes, F. necrophorum* or other bacteria produces an abscess in the heel or more commonly the toe of one claw. The abscess may burst out at the coronet or interdigital space.

Cinical signs
- Usually individual goats, involving one foot. The animal is very lame, often spending long periods lying down. There is considerable painful swelling of the affected claw, particularly in the interdigital space with bloody plus discharging between the digits or from the coronet.
- Pyrexia, anorexia.

Treatment
- Early treatment by paring to release the pus, bathing with antiseptic solution and poultice, together with systemic antibiotic therapy for about 10 days will be successful provided the deeper tissues and joints are not involved.
- Where the condition is more severe, considerable deformity of the foot may occur and amputation of the digit should be considered.

Orf (contagious pustular dermatitis)

Lesions of orf (qv) occasionally occur around the coronet or on the legs from licking and may result in lameness.

Strawberry footrot (mycotic dermatitis)

Dermatophilus congolense causes 'lumpy wool' and *Strawberry footrot* in sheep and goats. The incidence of both conditions appears to be very low in goats in the UK, although the condition is easily produced experimentally.

Initially there are raised (paint brush) tufts of hair followed by crusting with pus under the crusts. Removal of the crusts leaves circular, raised, red granulating lesions on the coronet interdigital space and lower leg as well as the body, scrotum and head. Lesions on the nose and ears must be distinguished from orf (qv) and those on the feet and lower leg from choroptic mange (qv). Predisposing conditions are wet, unhygienic conditions and ectoparasites which transfer zoospores between animals. Zoospores are generally carried in scabs between animals.

Diagnosis

Smears, skin biopsy or culture on blood agar.

Treatment

Dry conditions, broad spectrum antibiotics; topical applications of 10% zinc sulphate solution or 1% potash alum.

Foot-and-mouth disease

Foot-and-mouth disease produces vesicular lesions at the coronet, heel and interdigitally resulting in acute lameness, generally in all four feet. There are generally only occasional small lesions in the mouth but the teats may be affected. Other clinical signs include pyrexia, lethargy and anorexia.

Non-infectious disease of the foot

White line disease

Separation of the horn from the sensitive laminae at the white line is a common cause of lameness as the area becomes filled with dirt and debris with resulting pressure on the laminae. Early foot paring will quickly resolve the condition.

If infection occurs in the area, pus will collect and track to the coronary band forming a foot abscess (qv).

Bruising/trauma to the horn

Foreign body

Puncture of the sole by a foreign body such as a stone or nail results in immediate lameness in the affected leg and occasionally a goat is presented with a foreign body still embedded in the foot or interdigital area. If the foreign body is removed the penetration site opened up and drainage established, recovery will occur rapidly, but neglect may lead to abscess formation (qv).

Fracture of the distal phalanx

A fracture of the distal phalanx produces an acute lameness in one foot. Radiography is required to confirm the diagnosis. Resolution may occur if movement is restricted for at least 6 weeks by a waterproof plaster cast.

Laminitis (aseptic pododermatitis)

Aetiology

Laminitis is a metabolic disorder of the corium and germinal layer of the foot, produced by a degeneration of the vascular supply to the corium.

- *Acute laminitis* occurs in response to endotoxin release during ruminal acidosis or toxic conditions.
- *Subacute and subclinical laminitis* are produced by overfeeding over a longer period.
- *Chronic laminitis* develops where acute or subacute laminitis is not recognized or satisfactorily treated because horn formation is disturbed.
- Trauma to the hoof may also predispose to laminitis.
- A genetic predisposition may exist in some families.

Occurrence

Acute laminitis may occur:

- After any toxic condition such as mastitis, metritis, retained fetal membranes or pneumonia.
- A few days after kidding with or without one of the above conditions.
- As a sequel to acidosis
  in females fed high energy diets
  in silage fed goats with continued ingestion of acid silage.

Subacute and subclinical laminitis occurs:

- In goatlings and kids as young as 8 weeks where high protein/energy concentrate rations (together with inadequate fibre?) are fed.
- In does overfed for the level of production.
- In male goats fed on milking rations particularly during the summer months when they are not working. Mammary development and milk production in bucks, particularly British Saanens, or Saanens from high yielding families, is also accentuated at this time by overfeeding and there is a danger of mastitis developing.

Chronic laminitis occurs as a sequel to acute, subacute or subclinical laminitis.

Clinical signs

Acute laminitis – Sudden onset of tender foot or feet (generally both front feet but occasionally all four feet) with a disinclination to walk, prolonged recumbency or walking on knees and a shifting of weight distribution when standing to spare the affected feet, teeth grinding and other signs of pain, pyrexia, fall in milk yield. The coronet of the affected foot feels hot but the toe cold.

Subacute and subclinical laminitis are only differentiated by degree. In subacute laminitis minor gait abnormalities occur whereas in the subclinical condition no gait changes are present and the feet do not feel hot. *Subclinical laminitis is a common and underdiagnosed disease of dairy goats, particularly kids and goatlings, which leads to the development of hoof abnormalities in older animals.*

Haemorrhage of the wall, heel and particularly the sole is evident on routine foot trimming as fine reddish discoloration which, unlike bruising, is generally not painful.

As in cattle, subclinical laminitis leads to the development of other lamenesses because poor quality horn is produced with changes in horn growth particularly of the sole so that the shape of the claw is changed and there may be marked differences in height and width between the lateral and medial claws.

Chronic laminitis – The goat is chronically lame with a grossly deformed foot which may be extremely solid because of the failure to differentiate into wall and sole or very overgrown ('sledge runner foot'). In severe cases the wall and sole will loosen from the corium with concomitant downward rotation of the pedal bone (much rarer than in the horse). In Anglo Nubian goats, the front feet particularly may become extremely high ('platform soles') with very hard hoof material although the general shape of the foot remains fairly normal. These goats have a characteristic goose stepping walk and spend a lot of time on their knees.

Treatment and control

- Most cases of laminitis can be prevented by better manage-ment, particularly by correct feeding practice.
- Acute cases should be placed on a reduced protein/energy diet, i.e. hay and bran mashes with a very reduced concentrate ration and a deep bed provided. Antibiotic cover should be given to combat any infection or toxic cause of the condition together with a non-steroidal anti-inflammatory drug such as Flunixin meglamine (Finadyne, Schering Plough). Corticosteroids and antihistamines may be useful in early cases. Heat treatment of the feet will help restore the

circulation if used during the first few hours when vasoconstriction is occurring. Cold water treatment is of benefit later, and for about 7 days, to reduce the subsequent vasodilation.

- Chronic cases need careful foot trimming to relieve pain by reducing pressure on the sensitive areas. Regular repeat foot care is needed when the foot is grossly overgrown or mishapen.

Lameness above the foot

'Weak pasterns'

- Superficial digital flexor tendon weakness (Figure 6.1a).
- Superficial and deep digital flexor tendons, weak or ruptured (Figure 6.1b).
- Flexor tendons and suspensory ligament ruptured (Figure 6.1c).

'Weak pasterns' have been a longstanding problem in some families of dairy goats particularly among Saanens, British Saanens and their crosses. More recently, Angora goats imported from Tasmania and New Zealand have shown similar weaknesses. The condition would appear to be inherited as a recessive gene and be accentuated by inbreeding.

Weak pasterns produce excessive wear on the heels and a long foot with an overgrown toe.

Aetiology

- Weakness of the flexor tendons attached to the pastern joint, the degree of deformity depending on the degree of involvement of superficial digital flexor tendon, deep digital flexor tendon and the suspensory ligament (see Figure 6.1). Traumatic damage and rupture of the flexor tendons and suspensory ligament (see below) will produce similar conformational changes.

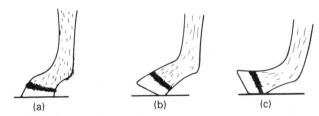

(a)   (b)   (c)

Figure 6.1 Weak pasterns

- The condition is accentuated by badly trimmed feet where the heels are cut short and the toes left long. Conversely well trimmed feet will ameliorate the condition to some extent. Poor trimming of the feet over a long period will produce the condition even in goats which are genetically sound.
- Older multiparous milking goats often show weakness of the superficial digital tendon.

Clinical signs

- Affected animals may show weakness by the time they are 6 months old with the condition worsening as the goat gets heavier through growth and pregnancy. Suspect animals will roll on their heels slightly, lifting the toe from the ground when encouraged to shift their weight backwards by pressing on the brisket. The hind legs are more commonly involved, but some goats show marked weakness in the front legs.

As the condition progresses, the joint adapts a characteristic right-angled bend because of weakness of the superficial flexor tendon with excessive wear on the heels. With the involvement of the deep flexor tendon the weight is shifted back onto the heels so the toes are raised from the ground, resulting in bruising to the heels. With complete collapse of the joint the weight is carried on the back of the foot without the sole touching the ground.

Accident or trauma
Fractures

Fractures of the limbs are more common in kids than adult goats (lameness in kids (qv)).

Soft tissue damage

A number of specific causes of lameness have been described.

(1) Rupture of the superficial and deep digital flexor tendons

Aetiology

- Trauma to the metacarpal or metatarsal region. A common cause of this injury is a tether becoming entangled around the leg and biting into the flesh – gross infection of the wound may be present as these cases are often neglected and severe restriction of the blood supply to the distal limb may lead to gangrene.

- Complete rupture of both flexor tendons produces a permanent unsoundness unless surgical repair is carried out. Severe lameness occurs and the animal is unwilling to bear weight as there is overflexion of the fetlock which touches the ground.
- A complete rupture of the superficial flexor tendon alone leads to slight lameness with a dropped fetlock and reasonable weight bearing.
- Incomplete rupture of the superficial tendon does not alter the ability to bear weight.

Treatment

- The wound should be thoroughly cleaned and the damage to the tendons assessed.
- Tendon repair can be carried out in a valuable animal using wire, carbon fibre or other suture material. The prognosis is good if only the superficial tendon is involved and poor if the deep tendon is damaged.
- The leg should be immobilized in a suitable external cast for at least a month.

(2) Rupture of the peroneus tertius muscle

Aetiology

- Trauma from a fall etc. results in rupture of the muscle, generally at its proximal origin on the stifle.

Clinical signs

- At rest, the limb is weight bearing, but there is a characteristic gait when walking with the foot dragged and the limb pulled backwards as the hock is extended with the stifle flexed and the Achilles tendon slack and loose.
- There is a painful swelling on the lateral side of the stifle.

Treatment and prognosis

- The prognosis is favourable, complete rest for about 6 weeks often resulting in recovery.

(3) Rupture of the cranial cruciate ligament

Aetiology

- Trauma to the stifle region.

Clinical signs

- During walking, the stifle is fixed with the heel raised from the ground and weight carried on the tip of the toe. A positive drawer forward sign is present.

Treatment

- Surgical treatment is essential or secondary damage to the joint may result in permanent lameness. Similar procedures to those used in the dog are satisfactory.

(4) Luxating patella

Generally the result of a congenital condition and obvious in the young goat but occasionally the result of trauma when luxation is generally medial.

(5) Radial nerve injury

Aetiology

- Trauma in the area of the upper limb or axilla.
- Lateral recumbency on a hard surface, e.g. during anaesthesia.

Clinical signs

- Dropped elbow with flexion of the carpus and fetlock.
- The foot is dragged as the carpus and fetlock cannot be extended.

Treatment

- Corticosteroids and diuretics to reduce the swelling around the nerve.
- Tendon transplantation has been used when the nerve injury was permanent.

Lameness after injection

Temporary lameness in goats is common after injections with irritant substances, e.g. tetracyclines, because of the relatively small muscular masses in the hind leg, particularly in the gluteal region. A more permanent lameness may result from damage to the sciatic or peroneal nerves. Because of the dangers involved in injecting into the limbs, the mid neck region has been recommended as a more suitable injection site.

Lameness may also be produced by painful swellings following the subcutaneous injection of irritant drugs (e.g. some oil adjuvanted vaccines) behind the elbow.

Sciatic nerve injury

Aetiology

- Injections in the gluteal muscle mass.

Clinical signs

- Loss of function in almost all of the hind limb with loss of skin sensation on the lateral surface of the tibial region and the hock and below.
- The foot is dragged. With each step the leg is pulled upward and forward by contraction of the quadriceps muscles which are innervated by the femoral nerve.

Treatment and prognosis

- Even severe cases may resolve but the prognosis is guarded.

Peroneal nerve injury

Aetiology

- Injections in the caudal thigh region.
- Trauma to the lateral surface of the thigh.

Clinical signs

- Paralysis of the muscles flexing the hock and extending the digits so that when the foot is brought forward there is knuckling at the fetlock and the hoof is dragged along the ground. If the foot is placed in position, normal weight bearing can occur.

Treatment and prognosis

- Prognosis is generally favourable with some improvement being seen in about a week.
- Anti-inflammatory drugs and diuretics will reduce swelling in the area of the nerve.
- In cases of permanent injury the fetlock joint can be ankylosed.

Carpal hygroma

Aetiology

- Persistent trauma to the carpal area results in the development of a bursa.
- Part of the caprine arthritis encephalitis syndrome (qv).

Clinical signs

- A firm non-painful swelling, often bilateral, on the dorsal aspect of the carpal joint.
- The animal is generally not lame.

Treatment

- Acute lesions may resolve without treatment but chronic conditions are unlikely to resolve.
- Aspiration of the bursal fluid may introduce infection if aseptic precautions are not carefully followed and is likely to produce only a temporary reduction in size.
- Injection with Lugol's iodine will destroy the membrane of the bursa.
- Surgical removal of the bursal sac can be undertaken for cosmetic reasons.

Osteopetrosis

Excessive calcium intake causing deposition in the bones and lameness in bucks and older does has been reported from the USA where large amounts of alfalfa hay is fed. In the UK where grass hay is normally fed, osteopetrosis is unlikely to present a problem.

Degenerative arthritis (osteoarthritis)

Aetiology

- A non-infectious arthritis resulting from degenerative changes in articular cartilage, together with hypertrophy of cartilage and bone.

Clinical signs

- A chronic lameness of gradual onset in older animals. The joints most commonly affected are the carpus, elbow, hock and stifle and these joints may be palpably enlarged with crepitus evident on manipulation.

- The goat may have difficulty rising or if only one leg is affected may continuously rest the limb.
- With lack of use, muscle wasting of the affected limb may be evident.

Treatment

- The response to anti-inflammatory drugs and analgesics such as phenylbutazone or corticosteroids is often disappointing and will often only provide temporary relief if any.

Caprine arthritis encephalitis (CAE)

- CAE is a disease of major importance in many parts of the world including France, Australia and the USA. In the UK estimates of the level of infection range from 4 to 8% and there are only a few reported clinical cases. Since 1983, many goatkeepers have been regularly blood testing for the virus and have adopted suitable control measures thus drastically limiting the spread of the disease. However, failure to maintain control measures could rapidly lead to an increased incidence of infection.

Aetiology

- A lentivirus, caprine arthritis encephalitis virus exists as a dominant DNA provirus in circulating monocytes. The virus is closely related to Maedi-Visna virus in sheep.

Transmission

- Through the colostrum or milk of infected does. The practice of feeding milk pooled from several does will facilitate spread of the disease throughout the kid population.
- By direct contact between goats, although prolonged contact is probably necessary, by virus shed in body fluids such as saliva, urogenital secretions, faeces and/or respiratory tract secretions.
- By transfer of blood from an infected to a non-infected goat, e.g. by tattooing or multiple use of needles.
- *In-utero* transmission probably does not occur.
- The virus is very labile in the environment and transmission via pasture or buildings, etc. will not occur.
- Direct cross species transmission between sheep and goats has not been demonstrated but lambs infected by goats' milk become infected with the virus and sheep inoculated with

virus experimentally became infected and developed lesions
of the disease.
- Goats infected with CAE remain virus carriers for life and
many symptomless carriers exist in the population. The virus
can thus be unwittingly spread throughout the flock or herd,
particularly to the young stock, without the owners being
aware of a carrier being present.

Clinical Signs

- Many goats remain symptomless carriers of the virus.
- The disease occurs in four clinical forms.

Arthritis

- Generally seen only in yearlings or adult goats although
occasionally in kids as young as 6 months.
- CAE virus affects all synovial membranes including those of
joints tendons and bursae and produces a chronic, progressive synovitis and arthritis with excess synovial fluid.
- Afebrile.
- Good appetite.
- Variable lameness, varying from slight stiffness to extreme
pain on standing.
- Gradual loss of condition depending on the degree of
lameness.
- The carpal (knee) joints are primarily affected and may be
grossly enlarged.
- Any other joint may be affected particularly the shoulder,
stifle, hock and fetlock and the atlantal and supraspinous
bursae are often enlarged later in the course of the disease.
- The course of the disease is variable, some animals merely
showing slight lameness for a number of years, others
showing an acute onset rapidly progressing restriction of
movement.

Hard udder
See Chapter 12.

Pneumonia
See Chapter 16.

Encephalitis
See Chapter 16.

Laboratory confirmation

(1) Serology
- Virus carriers are identified using an agar gel immunodiffusion test (AGIDT) or an enzyme linked immunosorbent assay (ELISA) to detect antibody to CAE. Antigens prepared from either CAE or Maedi-visna viruses can be used in these tests.
- The antibodies detected are not protective against disease, merely an indicator of infection, as only very low levels of neutralizing antibodies are produced in response to infection.
- Any goat which is seropositive on a CAE test is infected for life. Infection persists even in the presence of neutralizing antibodies because of the ability of the virus to exist as latent proviral DNA.

Conversely, however, a goat which is tested seronegative cannot be assumed free from infection, because: (i) current tests are relatively insensitive; (ii) the period between infection with the virus and seroconversion (i.e. production of detectable antibody) may be prolonged. Goats infected by contact or by drinking infected milk when adults may take 3 or more years to become seropositive. Kids infected postnatally generally seroconvert between 6 months and 1 year of age. Some seropositive goats will periodically test seronegative.

- Many goats seroconvert after a period of stress or at parturition. Testing in late pregnancy will not necessarily detect all does which seroconvert after kidding and these animals will produce infected kids.
- Kids which have received infected colostrum, have detectable levels of colostral antibody for 2 or 3 months but will subsequently test negative until they seroconvert and produce their own antibodies several months or even years later.
- Antibody levels may fall as the disease progresses so even a clinically diseased animal may test seronegative.
- More sensitive tests are available in specialized laboratories but not for routine screening.
  - (i)   Virus isolation.
  - (ii)   Detection of viral nucleic acid – polymerase chain reaction (PCR).
  - (iii) Western blotting – sensitive test for antibody detection.

The use of these more sensitive tests in the future may lead to the ability to detect latently-infected animals thus greatly facilitating eradication programmes.

Gross postmortem findings – joints

- Hyperplasia of synovial membranes with thickening, fibrosis and in chronic cases, calcification of joint capsule, tendons and ligaments.
- Periosteal reaction with periarticular osteophyte production.
- Degenerative joint disease with ulceration and erosion of the articular cartilages and destruction of subchondral bone.

(2) *Examination of synovial fluid:* reddish brown with large numbers of cells 1000–2000/ mm, mainly mononuclear cells (cf normal goats < 500 cells/ mm); may contain fibrin tags. Locally produced antibody may be detectable in the fluid.

(3) *Histological examination – joints*

- Subsynovial mononuclear cell infiltration and hyperplasia.
- Synovial villus hypertrophy.
- Focal areas of necrosis within the synovial membrane or surrounding connective tissue.

Diagnosis

Diagnosis should be based on:

- Serum antibody levels to CAE virus.
- Clinical signs.
- Postmortem lesions.
- Histopathological change.
- Virus isolation from synovial or brain cells.
- Radiology may aid in determining the severity or progression of arthritic lesions in individual animals and demonstrate pneumonia.

Treatment

- There is no treatment at present for CAE.
- Non-steroidal anti-inflammatory drugs such as flunixin meglamine (Finadyne, Schering Plough) and phenylbutazone can be used to relieve the pain of arthritis.

Prevention and control

- Routine tests at 6-monthly to yearly intervals for a minimum of 5 years and preferably more with no evidence of infection in the herd during that time are required before a herd can be said to be 'CAE virus free'.
- No kid should receive unpasteurized goats' milk or colostrum from any animal except its dam. Pooled milk should *never* be fed to kids. If a doe subsequently proves to be a virus carrier only her own kids will have been infected.
- All adult goats (or in the case of a kid, its dam) should be blood tested before entry into the herd.
- No milk from another herd should be fed under any circumstances.

The infected herd/flock

- Cull or isolate all reactors.
- Cull or isolate the offspring of all reactors.
- Infected goats should be separated from non-infected goats by at least 1.8 m. Separate feeding/water utensils should be used.
- Milk infected goats last; keep milk separate from any non-infected milk used for feeding kids.
- As the virus is labile in the environment, infected goats can graze the same pastures as non-infected goats provided the groups are kept separate, i.e. graze non-infected goats in the morning and infected in the afternoon.
- Because the incidence of uterine infection by the virus is very low, removing the kids at birth from reactors by 'snatching', i.e. preventing suckling or licking by the dam enables a non-infected kid to be produced in the vast majority of cases.
- Batch mate and induce parturition using prostaglandins (qv) or delay parturition by use of Planipart (Boehringer Ingelheim).
- Isolate kids, house separately from infected goats, and rear on cows' colostrum and milk or calf or kid milk replacer. If goats' milk or colostrum is fed it must be pasteurized even if it comes from a supposedly seronegative doe. Milk can be pasteurized by heating for one hour at 56°C but this will *not* ensure 100% death of the virus and pasteurized milk from known carriers should never be fed. Haemolysis very occasionally occurs in kids fed cows' milk (see Chapter 18). The dangers from producing kids with low colostral

anitbiodies must be weighed against the possible dangers of CAE infection in each herd.

- Blood sample kids shortly after birth to detect any possible passive transfer of antibody if the snatching was not done efficiently, then at 6 months and at 3-monthly intervals thereafter to detect possible virus carriers.

Control schemes

- Individual herd scheme – tailored to control the disease within one herd along the lines previously described.
- British Goat Society Monitored Herd Scheme – a scheme for monitoring the disease status of goat herds by testing but with no restrictions on the movement of goats.
- MAFF Sheep/Goat Health Scheme – monitors the disease status of the herd by regular blood tests and by restricting movement between herds aims to maintain herds as CAE free.

Further reading

General

Adams, D. S. (1983) Infectious causes of lameness above the foot. *Vet. Clin. North Amer.: Large Animal Practice*, 5 (3), Nov. 1983 499–510

Cottom, D. S. and Pinsent, P. J. N. (1988) Lameness in the goat. *Goat Vet. Soc. J.*, 9 (1/2), 14–23

Merrall, M. (1985) Lameness in goats. In *Proc. of a Course in Goat Husbandry and Medicine*. Massey University, November 1985, Publ. No. 106, 66–77

Nelson, D. R. (1983) Non-infectious causes of lameness above the foot. *Vet. Clin. North Amer.: Large Animal Practice*, 5 (3), Nov 1983 491–498

Smith, M. C. (1983) Foot problems in goats. *Vet. Clin. North Amer.: Large Animal Practice*, 5 (3), No. 1983 489–490

Footrot

Hay, L. A. (1990) Footrot and related conditions. *Goat Vet. Soc. J.*, II (1), 1–6

Arthritis

Smith, J. *et al.* (1989) Drug therapy for arthritis in food producing animals. *Comp. Cont. Ed. Pract. Vet.*, II (1), 89–93

Caprine arthritis encephalitis

Adams, D. S. *et al.* (1983) Transmission and control of CAE virus. *Am. J. Vet. Res.*, 44 (9), 1670–1675

Dawson, M. (1987) Caprine arthritis encephalitis. *In Practice*, Jan. 1987, 8–11

Knight, A. P. and Jokinen, M. P. (1982) Caprine arthritis encephalitis. *Comp. Cont. Ed. Pract. Vet.*, 4 (6), S263–S269

7 Lameness in kids

Trauma
Congenital abnormalities
Infections
Nutritional

Trauma

Congenital abnormalities

- Overextension of the stifle and hock.
- Contracted tendons.
- Angular limb deformities and arthrogryposis.
- Luxation of the patella.

Infections

- Joint ill.
- Tick pyaemia .
- Mycoplasma.
- Chlamydia.
- Erysipelas.
- Other bacterial arthritides.
- Footrot/interdigital dermatitis.

Nutritional.

- Calcium, phosphorus and vitamin D deficiency or imbalance
  Angular limb deformities
  Rickets
  Osteodystrophia fibrosa.
- White muscle disease.
- Copper deficiency.

Trauma

- 'The kid is an accident waiting to happen'
  The most common lamenesses in kids are the result of
  accident or trauma, resulting in bruising, sprains, strains or
  fractures particularly of the front legs.

Fractures

Occur most frequently in the metacarpal region followed by the
radius/ulna, tibia and metatarsus. In many cases, palpation
permits identification of the site of the fracture but radiography
may be required for confirmation if there is little bone
displacement.

External fixation with plaster or lightweight resin material is extremely well tolerated. If necessary internal fixation, using pin or plate, can be undertaken using techniques similar to that used in the dog. Where possible additional external support is indicated because of the robust use of the leg which will occur as the fracture heals.

Foreign bodies

e.g. thorns, may penetrate the hoof more easily in kids than adult goats.

Congenital abnormalities

Overextension of the stifle and hock

Aetiology

- Overextension of the hock and stifle is common in newly born kids and is usually bilateral, although one leg is often more severely effected than the other.

Clinical signs

- The kid has difficulty walking as the leg tends to bow and the stifle and hock joints are unstable.

Treatment

- No treatment is generally necessary as the condition normally corrects itself within a few days, but it is necessary to ensure that the kid is mobile enough to suckle adequately from its dam.

Contracted tendons

Congenital, bilateral contraction of the flexor tendons of the forelimbs is common and results in flexion of the fetlocks so that the animal walks on its fetlocks or with partially flexed fetlocks.

Treatment

- Mild cases with only partial flexion of the fetlocks will resolve on their own as the tendons stretch with movement.
- More severe cases may need splinting to stretch the tendons and allow weight bearing on the foot.

Angular limb deformities and arthrogryposis

Congenital limb deformities involving the bones and joints are occasionally seen in newborn goats and generally result in a bilateral articular rigidity, particularly flexion of phalangeal, metacarpo-phalangeal and carpal joints.

Treatment

- Cases of mild articular rigidity may correct themselves with weight bearing. Surgical treatment of severe retractions can be attempted in valuable animals.

Luxation of the patella

Aetiology

- Lateral luxation of the patella is an uncommon problem in goats and is usually congenital. Anglo Nubian goats are more prone to the condition because of the upright conformation of their hind legs. In Swiss breeds, luxation occasionally occurs as the result of acute trauma in the adult goat and is generally *medial*.

Clincal signs

- The luxation may be bilateral or unilateral, permanent or intermittent. In its severest form, the stifles will remain permanently flexed, so that the animal adopts a crouching stance and has difficulty standing. Where the condition is intermittent there will be periods of acute lameness which is relieved when the patella is returned to the normal position by manipulation.

Treatment

- Mild intermittent luxation requires no treatment, more severe luxations can be corrected surgically and severe congential luxations may necessitate euthanasia.

Infections

Joint ill

A bacterial arthritis of young kids under 3 months of age.

Aetiology

- A number of bacteria may be involved. These are usually environmental contaminants, particularly haemolytic *Streptococcus* spp. and *Staphylococcus* spp. but also *Corynebacterium* spp. and *E. coli* etc. Infection occurs through the umbilical cord shortly after birth.

Clinical signs

- Pain and swelling in one or more joints of a neonatal kid, especially carpus, shoulder, hock and stifle. Occasionally pronounced lameness with minimum joint swelling. In more chronic cases, the affected joint will be stiff or even ankylosed.
- The kid may or may not be pyrexic depending on the stage and type of infection.
- The umbilicus is often inflamed.

Laboratory investigation

- Joint fluid or umbilical swabs can be cultured for bacteria if indicated.

Control and treatment

- A clean environment at kidding.
- Treat umbilical cord with Lugol's iodine or antibiotic spray as soon after birth as possible and then check regularly for signs of inflammation or infection.
- Adequate colostrum, i.e. about 300 ml within 6 hours of birth.
- Broad spectrum antibiotics parenterally and intra-articularly but the response to treatment is often poor.
- Intra-articular lavage may remove pus and reduce damage to the joint surfaces.

Tick pyaemia (enzootic staphylococcal infection)

Aetiology

- *Staphylococcus aureus;* the tick *Ixodes ricinus* damages the kid's skin permitting penetration of the bacteria which are already present on the skin surface.
- Infection with tickborne fever (qv) may exacerbate the pathogenicity of tick pyaemia.

Clinical signs

- Variable depending on the sites of abscesses which form in various parts of the body, e.g. liver, spinal cord, following the introduction of the bacteria and the resulting pyaemia.
- Hot swollen painful joints (particularly carpal joints and hocks); lameness; eventually chronic arthritis with permanent lameness and poor growth rates.
- Various neurological signs – blindness, incoordination, posterior paraplegia.

Treatment

- Early cases can be treated with penicillin.
- Superficial abscesses can be lanced and drained.
- Once severe joint lesions are present, treatment is not successful.

Mycoplasma

Mycoplasma spp. have been reported to cause arthritis in goats (usually kids under 6 months) in Europe, Australia and the USA and with increasing numbers of goats being imported into the UK, mycoplasma should be regarded as a possible importation hazard.

Aetiology

Mycoplasma spp. such as *M. capricolum*, and *M. mycoides* subsp. *mycoides*.

Clinical signs

- Outbreaks of arthritis generally in kids and young goats with acutely swollen joints and pyrexia with or without pneumonia.

Postmortem findings

- Purulent or fibropurulent arthritis with haemorrhagic erosions of articular surfaces.
- Lungs collapsed and rubbery.

Diagnosis

- Serology (CFT).
- Isolation of the organism from joint fluid in mycoplasma medium.

Chlamydia

Chlamydia psittaci has been reported to cause polyarthritis in young goats in parts of Europe and the USA but not in the UK, although the organism has been isolated from sheep joints in this country.

Clincal signs

- Polyarthritis and stiffness as part of an acute febrile illness in a number of kids.

Postmortem findings

- Fibrinous arthritis with no changes to the cartilage.

Diagnosis

- Smears of joint exudate stained with Giemsa.
- Immunofluorescence.
- Isolation of chlamydia in embryonating yolk sacs.

Erysipelas

Erysipelas polyarthritis has been occasionally reported in kids under 2 months of age.

Aetiology

- The bacterium *Erysipelothrix insidiosa* enters through breaks in the skin, e.g. castration wounds, or via the umbilicus.

Clinical signs

- Pyrexia, anorexia and lethargy with hot swollen painful joints in the acute stage. The disease often becomes chronic.

Diagnosis

- Isolation of the organism from joints in acute cases.

Treatment

- High doses of penicillin.

Other bacterial arthritides

Other bacteria may occasionally cause arthritis either as a result of septicaemia or direct penetration into the joint from a puncture wound.

Footrot/interdigital dermatitis

See Chapter 6. Infection with *Fusobacterium necrophorum* and *Bacteroides nodosus* may become significant in older kids.

Nutritional

Calcium, phosphorus and vitamin D deficiency or imbalance

- Kids are susceptible to imbalances in the calcium:phosphorus ratio. The calcium:phosphorus ratio in goat diets should not drop below 1.2:1 and should ideally be around 2:1.
- Vitamin D is essential for the absorption and metabolism of calcium and phosphorus.
- On typical diets in the UK a relative calcium deficiency is more likely than a calcium excess.

Angular limb deformities

Angular limb deformities may be present at birth (qv) but mild limb deformities are also the commonest manifestation of calcium:phosphorus imbalance in goats in the UK.

Aetiology

- Acquired limb deformities occur in a rapidly growing early maturing kid with a calcium:phosphorus imbalance.
- Angulation of the limb results in epiphyseal compression producing increased pressure on the growth plate on that side and retarding growth.

Clinical signs

- Outward (lateral) deviation of the fetlock joint (fetlock valgus) is the commonest deformity seen in young goats, but more severe imbalances may result in knock knees (carpal valgus) or carpal and stifle varus (bow legs).
- Uneven wear of the feet may occur.
- Lameness.

Treatment

- Correct dietary imbalances.
- Use corrective foot trimming on a fortnightly basis.
- The application of splints in the early stages of carpal varus and fetlock valgus may correct the problem.
- Surgical compression of the growth plate with staples or screws and wire will slow the growth on that side and allow the limb to straighten. Early remedial action is necessary before the natural closure of the growth plates.

Rickets

Rickets is a disease of young growing kids characterized by defective calcification of growing bone.

Aetiology

Relative or absolute dietary deficiencies of calcium, phosphorus and vitamin D. Rapidly growing kids kept indoors on an otherwise good diet are most likely to be affected.

Clinical signs

- Enlarged painful epiphyses and costochondral junctions.
- Poor appetite and unthriftiness.
- Stiff gait, lameness, unwillingness to stand.
- Arched back.
- Possible bending of the long bones.

Prevention

- Exercise in sunlight with increased vitamin D levels.
- Feed sun-dried hay.
- Calcium and phosphorus supplements where necessary.
- Vitamin D 500 i.u. or Vitamins A, D and E 125,000 i.u.

Treatment

- Correct any calcium/phosphorus imbalance with supplements as necessary.
- Vitamin D 500 i.u. injection.

Daily calcium/phosphorus requirements

	Gain g/day	Calcium (g)	Phosphorus (g)
Maintenance			
50 kg		2.5	1.5
80 kg		4.0	2.4
Production requirements/kg milk		4.0	3.0
Gestation requirements last 2 months		1.5	1.8
Kid daily requirements			
1 m	175	2.0	1.3
2 m	200	2.7	1.7
3–5 m	175	2.9	1.9
6 m	150	3.2	2.0

(After Tomas, G. S. and Turner, W. J. (1979)
Quoted in Baxendell, S. A. (1984)).

Osteodystrophia fibrosa

Aetiology

- Like rickets, osteodystrophia fibrosa is caused by imbalance of calcium and phosphorus and results from a secondary calcium deficiency due to excess phosphorus feeding, giving a calcium:phosphorus ratio of 1:2.5 or greater.
- Cereals and bran are high in phosphorus. Diets low in fresh green food and good hay but high in cereals and bran, predispose to the disease.

Clinical signs

- Unthriftiness.
- Poor appetite.
- Lameness.
- Bilateral swelling of bones of the face and jaw.
- Molar and premolar teeth rotated and loose.
- Fractures of long bones.
- Bones soft.

Prevention and treatment

- Correct the calcium:phosphorus ratio in the ration.
- Feed diet high in green foods; add bonemeal or powdered limestone.
- Severely affected animals with distorsion of the mandible should be culled.

White muscle disease

Vitamin E and selenium both have antioxidant functions and can partially substitute for one another in the diet. Vitamin E requirements of the goat may be higher than those of sheep and cattle.

Aetiology

- A selenium/Vitamin E deficiency produces a degenerative myopathy, particularly in very young kids born to deficient dams. The clinical signs depend on whether the skeletal muscles (skeletal muscle form) or the heart muscle and diaphragm (cardiac form) are affected or both forms may appear together in the same animal.

Predisposing conditions

- Selenium deficient pastures, where animals are fed on locally produced feed without supplementation.
- Vitamin E deficient diets – poor quality hay or straw with little concentrate.
- High levels of unsaturated fatty acids, e.g. fish/soya oils, calf milk with added vegetable fat causes relative vitamin E deficiency.

Clinical signs

- Kids are affected at birth or up to 6 months of age but generally between 2 and 16 weeks. The most active kids are often affected first and the disease is often seen 2–3 days after turnout.

(1) Skeletal muscle form

- Stiffness and reluctance to move; lie down frequently; stand up with difficulty; cry if forced to move.
- Skeletal muscles firm and painful on palpation (cf nervous disease) particularly in the hind limbs.
- Non-pyrexic.
- Appetite remains good even if the kid is unable to stand.

(2) Cardiac form

- Sudden death, typically in kids 2–6 months old after or during exercise.

- Tachycardia.
- Tachypnoea; hyperpnoea.
- Weakness.

Older kids and adults may show signs of the skeletal muscle form after stress or exercise.

Postmortem findings

- Pale or white streaks in the skeletal muscles, particularly of the hind limbs and lumbar area and the subendocardial muscle of the venticles of the heart.

Laboratory findings

- Creatine phosphokinase (CPK) and aspartate transaminase (AST) markedly elevated.
- Blood selenium levels below 50 ppb (normal 158–160 ppb; marginal 50–80 ppb).
- Glutathione peroxidase levels low.
- Liver selenium levels below 500 nmol/kg or vitamin E below 2.5 μmol/kg considered deficient.

Prevention

- Inject the does with selenium/vitamin E one month before kidding and/or
- Inject the kids at birth and 3–4 weeks of age and possibly 12–16 weeks of age.
- Add selenium at 100 ppm to feed.
- Oral drenching with 5 mg sodium selenite during the last week of pregnancy.
- Oral drenching with selenium combined with anthelmintics.

Treatment

- Affected animals should be treated with a combined selenium/vitamin E preparation, e.g. Vitesel (Norbrook Laboratories) or Dystosel (Intervet) 0.5–1.0 ml.

NB *Selenium toxicity*: Overdosage with selenium supplements may result in selenium poisoning. Acute poisoning produces dyspnoea, diarrhoea, pyrexia, tachycardia, apparent blindness, head pressing, collapse and death. Chronic poisoning may occur with long-term supplementation or in parts of the world with naturally high selenium levels in the soil but is unlikely to occur in the UK – lethargy, weight loss, pica, lameness, neurological signs.

Copper deficiency

The ataxia produced by copper deficiency (sway back or enzootic ataxia (qv) may be confused with lameness in kids from birth to 4 weeks of age.

Further reading

General

See Chapter 6.

Baxendell, S. A (1984) Caprine limb and joint conditions. *Proc. Univ. Sydney Post. Grad. Common Vet. Sci.* **73**, 370

8 Chronic weight loss in goats

Initial assessment
Clinical examination
Primary nutritional deficiency
Inability to utilize available foodstuffs
Unwillingness to utilize available foodstuffs
Inability to increase feed intake to match
production demands
Interference with absorption of nutrients/loss
of nutrients
Interference with rumen/intestinal mobility
Presence of chronic disorders
Pruritic conditions

Primary nutritional deficiency

- Starvation
    neglect
    inexperience
- Trace element deficiency
    cobalt
    copper
    Vitamin E/selenium

Inability to utilize available foodstuffs

- Dentition.
- Mouth lesions.
- Facial paralysis.
- Lameness.
- Blindness.
- Bullying.

Unwillingness to utilize available foodstuffs

- Male goats at the start of the breeding season.
- Unpalatable feed – spoilage, mould etc.
- Change in feed.

Inability to increase feed intake to match production demands

- Peak lactation.
- Periparturient toxaemia (pregnancy toxaemia, postparturient toxaemia, ketosis, acetonaemia).

Interference with absorption of nutrients/loss of nutrients

- Gastrointestinal parasitizm.
- Johne's disease (paratuberculosis).
- Liver disease
    chronic fascioliasis
    abscess

tumour
ragwort poisoning
visceral cysticercosis
hydatid disease.

Interference with rumen/intestinal mobility

- Chronic rumen impaction.
- Ascites – chronic fascioliasis.
- Ruminoreticular ulceration.
- Adhesions following surgery.
- Tumour – carcinomas.
- Cestode infection?
- Left-sided displacement of the abomasum.

Presence of chronic diseases

- Pneumonia
    pasteurella
    CAE
    Lungworm infection
    Viruses
    (mycoplasma)
    (caseous lymphadenitis).
- Peritonitis.
- Enteritis.
- Mastitis.
- Metritis.
- Tuberculosis.

Pruritic conditions

- Lice.
- Sarcoptic mange.
- Scrapie.

Initial assessment

Consider

- Individual or herd/flock problem.
- Similar cases in the herd in the past.

- Management practices.
   housing/availability of shelter/general hygiene
   feeding systems
   size of groups; age mix of groups; recent mixing of goats?
   horned/disbudded goats
   grazing history
   routine medication – worming, external parasite control.
- Stage of lactation/pregnancy.
- Milk yield.

Clinical examination

- Body condition – *condition scoring* of dairy goats is difficult as most of the body fat is carried internally. Apparently thin, bony goats may be found to have a large amount of abdominal fat at postmortem. With Angora goats, scoring is slightly easier but never so accurate as with cattle or sheep.
   Score 1. Very lean: body angular; lumbar vertebrae prominent with transverse processes readily palpable.
   Score 2. Lean: lumbar vertebrae less prominent, transverse processes easily palpated but with some tissue cover.
   Score 3. Good condition: lumbar vertebrae and transverse processes palpable but with reasonable cover; moderately rounded appearance to body.
   Score 4. Fat: lumbar vertebrae only palable with gentle pressure and the transverse processes with firm pressure, body smooth and rounded.
   Condition score 2 is adequate during lactation with condition rising to score 3 at the time of service.
- *Regular weighing* is the most accurate way of monitoring condition in a particular flock or herd.
- General examination at rest to include skin (lice, mange), mouth (teeth, lesions), feet (footrot, laminitis), mucous membranes (anaemia), abdomen (ascites, rumen function), auscultation of thorax (cardiac/respiratory function), lymph nodes.

Primary nutritional deficiency

Starvation

Failure to ensure that the ration provides adequate energy and protein to meet the needs of maintenance, growth and production, together with sufficient minerals and vitamins and clean water.

- Neglect.
- Inexperience
    inappropriate feedstuffs
    unbalanced ration
    feed shortage at critical times.

Daily requirements for energy and protein

Maintenance (80 kg goat)	10 MJ +	6.5 g DCP
Plus milk/litre (3.5% BF)	5.19 MJ + 48	g DCP
Pregnancy (average last 2 months)	6.0 MJ + 54	g DCP
Mohair production (6.0 kg/annum)	0.75 MJ + 18	g DCP

Obvious dietary deficiencies can generally be easily remedied. Less obvious problems can be investigated by analysing feedstuffs or by *metabolic profiles* of a number of goats in the herd.
Suggested profiles are:

- Energy: Glucose, β hydroxybutyrate, non-esterified fatty acids, ketones.
- Protein: Total protein, albumen, urea.
- Trace element: Copper, zinc, iron, selenium, cobalt.

Trace element deficiency

(1) *Cobalt deficiency (pine)*

Aetiology

- Primary deficiency of cobalt in the diet produces signs of vitamin B_{12} deficiency with inability to metabolize propionic acid.
- A secondary B_{12} deficiency may occur with helminth infection.

Incidence

- Certain areas of the UK are known to be cobalt deficient.

Laboratory tests

- Blood cobalt or vitamin B_{12} levels are a poor guide to cobalt status (suggested that 150–300 pmol B_{12}/l) is considered marginal and over 300 pmol B_{12}/l adequate).

- Liver cobalt and vitamin B_{12} levels provide useful guide (normal cobalt levels 0.2–0.3 ppm DM).
- <0.1 ppm DM cobalt on pasture sample suggests cobalt deficiency.
- The presence in urine of methylmalonic acid (MMA) and forminoglutamic acid (FIGLU) indicates cobalt deficiency.

Clinical signs
- Growing animal more severely affected than the adult.
- Unthriftiness.
- Inappetence.
- Wasting.
- Emaciation.
- Ocular discharge.
- Anaemia (normocytic, normochromic).
- Reduced milk production.
- Death.

Diagnosis
- Response to cobalt or B_{12}.

Treatment and control
- B_{12} injections (100 mg/week).
- Cobalt (7 mg/week), administered as cobalt oxide bullets (Permaco-S, Coopers Pitman-Moore) or in the water (Aqua-trace Cobalt tablets, Denis Brinicombe) or as a drench (Copacobal, C-Vet).
- Cobalt sulphate applied as a top dressing to pasture every 3 or 4 years (2 kg/ha).

(2) *Copper deficiency*

As well as neurological signs (see Chapter 15) copper deficiency may result in growth retardation, emaciation, microcytic anaemia, diarrhoea and increased susceptibility to infection.

(3) *Selenium deficiency* (see white muscle disease)

May occasionally cause illthrift.

Inability to utilize available foodstuffs

Dentition

Goats over 5 years of age kept extensively show increasing wear of the incisor and molar teeth, so prehension and mastication may become difficult.

Uneven wear of molar teeth can result in sharp points leading to ulceration of the buccal cavity and tongue, often complicated by secondary bacterial infections – goats may show reluctance to eat, chewing on one side and pouching or dropping of food. Congenital defects such as overshot/undershot jaws may predispose to dental problems.

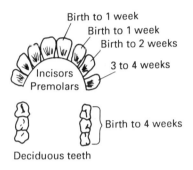

Deciduous teeth

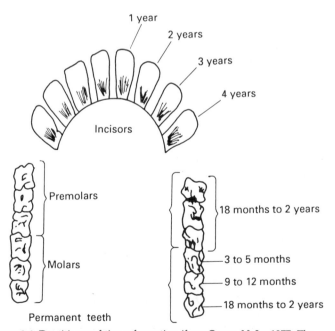

Figure 8.1 Dentition and time of eruption (from Owen, N. L., 1977, *The Illustrated Standard of the Dairy Goat*, Dairy Goat Journal Publishing Corporation)

Mouth lesions

Painful mouth lesions from infection (e.g. Orf (qv)), toxic material resulting in mouth ulceration (e.g. giant hogweed poisoning), necrotic stomatitis from eating abrasive plant material, drenching given injuries or perodontal disease will inhibit eating.

Facial paralysis

e.g. listeriosis (qv).

Lameness (see Chapters 6 and 7)

Lameness will reduce grazing or feeding at troughs if the pain is severe. In particular:

- Chronic degenerative joint disease – CAE, osteoarthritis etc.
- Footrot or interdigital dermatitis.
- Laminitis.
- Overgrown feet.

Blindness (see Chapter 19)

- Severe keratoconjunctivitis.
- Vitamin A deficiency.
- Post CCN.
- (Lead).

Bullying

Goats have a well established rigid social order – the bottom goat(s) may be denied access to food.
The problem may be precipitated by:

- Introducing a new goat into an established group.
- Providing insufficient space/goat (3.3–9.3 m^2/goat).
- Providing insufficient trough space (0.4–0.6 m/goat).
- Having groups of mixed ages.
- Running horned goats with polled or disbudded goats.

Unwillingness to utilize available feedstuffs

- Male goats at the start of the breeding season will often refuse feed with consequent weight loss.

- Unpalatable feed – spoilage, mould etc. Goats will refuse unwholesome feed.
- Even a change in food, e.g. a batch of concentrates may result in feed refusal for a week or more.

Inability to increase feed intake to match production demands

Peak lactation

All heavily lactating goats, particularly young first kidders will lose weight despite the availability of an adequate diet. On a body weight for weight basis, goats are much heavier producers than cows. 'Running through' these milkers the following year (i.e. allowing a 2 year gap between kidding) allows time for these animals to regain their body reserves and prevents restriction of growth. In the second year of lactation, a good milker will give 80+% of its first year milk yield.

Periparturient toxaemia (pregnancy toxaemia, postparturient toxaemia, acetonaemia, ketosis)

Periparturient toxaemia occurs in response to insufficient intake of energy to meet the increasing demands of pregnancy or lactation.

(1) *Before kidding* – in the last 4–6 weeks of pregnancy as *pregnancy toxaemia* or
(2) *After kidding* – usually about 2–4 weeks postpartum. Most does suffer a mild ketonaemia in early lactation as the demands of the lactation for energy are not met adequately by the diet. In most animals an equilibrium is established and the ketosis remains subclinical. Goats which are not overfat may develop an acute clinical ketosis or *acetonaemia*. Goats, which have large fat deposits at kidding may develop a *postparturient toxaemia* similar to pregnancy toxaemia or fatty liver disease of cows, presumably in response to impaired liver function.

Predisposing factors

- Multiple fetuses
  (a) nutritional drain on dam during last 6 weeks of pregnancy

(b) compression of the rumen by fetuses decreases voluntary food intake. Suboptimum food intake is the main predisposing factor in periparturient toxaemia.
- Goat overfed as a goatling.
- Goat overfed during the dry period at the end of parturition
  (a) intra-abdominal fat deposits reduce the rumen capacity and thus food intake
  (b) excessive quantities of fat are mobilized from body depots and deposited in the liver; fatty infiltration of the liver results in hepatic dysfunction.
- Lack of exercise.
- Undernutrition – undoubtedly a major cause of pregnancy toxaemia and acetonaemia in goats kept extensively, through inadequate food supply, poorly balanced rations or heavy worm burdens but *not* a major cause of periparturient toxaemia in intensively kept dairy goats in the UK where most goats which show the disease are being offered an adequate balanced ration.
- Stress – stress factors (fear, weather, housing etc) play a part in initiating the disease in goats on a poor plane of nutrition, but in the majority of cases in dairy goats there is no obvious stress involved.

Laboratory tests

- Ketostix, Multistix, Acetest tablets or Rotheras reagent can be used to detect ketones in urine or milk.
- Blood sample can be submitted for an energy profile – glucose, β-hydroxybutyrate, non-esterified fatty acids, ketones
  Changes in liver enzyme levels are not generally useful for diagnosis.

Pregnancy toxaemia

Clinical signs

- Initially inappetence (eats browsings/hay, refuses concentrates) later complete anorexia.
- Lethargic, unwilling to move; walks with difficulty legs may swell.
- Weight loss.
- Occasionally nervous signs – tremor around the head and ears reduced vision or blindness, head pressing, stargazing eventually recumbency, coma with or without abortion, death.

Treatment

- In the absence of abortion or parturition, treatment is generally unsatisfactory. Terminate pregnancy by inducing parturition (qv) or caesarian section or rapid removal of kids by non-sterile caesarian section under local anaesthesia followed by euthanasia of the doe. Use dexamethasone rather than prostaglandins to induce parturition – improved survival of kids, plus gluconeogenic effect in the dam. Give calcium borogluconate because hypocalcaemia may coexist with the condition.

Postmortem findings

- Emaciated carcase or large amounts of abdominal fat.
- Yellow orange enlarged liver which is greasy and friable.
- Adrenal glands may be enlarged.

Postparturient toxaemia (fatty liver syndrome)

Clinical signs

- Inappetence (eats browsings/hay, refuses concentrates), later complete anorexia.

- Milk yield initially depressed and then drops markedly.
- Lethargic.
- Chronic weight loss over several weeks.
- Eventually recumbency, coma and death – most goatkeepers will request euthanasia before this stage is reached.

Postmortem findings

- As for pregnancy toxaemia.

Treatment

- Encourage the goat to continue eating (anything!) – usually best response to browsings, green food (e.g. ivy in winter). Goats which continue to eat may survive, totally anorexic animals will die.
- Stimulate appetite with products such as Rumen Stimulent (Univet), Restart (Bayer) and B vitamins.
- Provide glucogenic agents
  - (1) 200 ml of 20% glucose solution, part i.v. or i.p., the rest s.c.

(2) 60 ml of glycerine (glycerol) in warm water twice daily or propylene glycol (Ketol, Intervet) 200 ml twice daily for 4–5 days.

- Stimulate gluconeogenesis.
  (1) Dexamethasone 25 mg injection (will also produce abortion in late pregnancy)
  or
  (2) Dexamethasone + protamine zinc insulin (up to 40 i.u. s.c twice daily) – insulin has an antilipolytic effect as well as effecting peripheral glucose utilization.
  (3) Anabolic steroids.
- Supportive therapy.
  (1) Multivitamins – particularly A/D. Vitamin E/selenium preparations may help hepatic metabolism in postparturient toxaemia.
  (2) Electrolytes – 1 to 3 litres of a balanced electrolyte solution (plus bicarbonate if respiratory acidosis is present).
  (3) Calcium borogluconate 20% with magnesium and phosphorus – 80–100 ml i.v. or s.c. in case of concomitant hypocalcaemia.
  (4) Restoration of normal rumen microflora – use natural yoghurt or probiotics or drench rumen contents from healthy animal.

Acetonaemia

Clinical signs

- Inappetance (eats browsings/hay, refuses concentrates).
- Mild ataxia.
- Constipation.
- Acetone smell to breath.
- Milk yield drops.

Treatment

- Corticosteroids.
- Other treatments as for postparturient toxaemia.

Prognosis

- Good; animals with this form of ketosis respond well to treatment.

NB Left-sided displacement of the abomasum (see chapter 14) produces a secondary ketosis and clinical signs similar to primary acetonaemia.

Interference with absorption of nutrients/loss of nutrients

Gastrointestinal parasitism (qv)

Trichostrongylus spp – diarrhoea
Ostertagi ostertagi – illthrift ± diarrhoea
Haemonchus contortus – anaemia

- A major cause of chronic weight loss. All cases should be assumed to be infected until *proved* otherwise (consider underdosing with anthelmintics, dosing at incorrect time and resistance, particularly with Benzamidazole products).
- A single low faecal egg count is not sufficient to eliminate internal parasitizm as a cause of weight loss, as egg counts may not reliably indicate the number of adult worms present (see Chapter 13).

Johne's disease (paratuberculosis)

Aetiology

- Acidfast bacterium, *Mycobacterium paratuberculosis*

Epidemiology

- Excreted in faeces by clinically ill or symptomless carriers.
- Persists in environment for months.
- Some animals may be intermittent excretors.
- Kids generally infected in first few weeks of life by faecal contamination of the udder or environment or possibly through infected colostrum (intrauterine transmission and infection via semen have also been demonstrated in cattle).
- Ingested organisms remain dormant in the gastrointestinal tract and adjacent lymph nodes, often for many years.
- Clinical disease may be precipitated by stress such as parturition or introduction to a new herd.

Clinical signs

- Adult goats, generally 3 + years.
- Progressive weight loss, lethargy.
- Decreased milk yield, loss of fibre.
- Diarrhoea generally only in the terminal stages.
- Anaemia – signs may be complicated by concomitant disease, e.g. CAE or respiratory disease.

Diagnosis

- Very difficult in the living animal and generally considered to be grossly underdiagnosed.
- Identification of the acidfast organisms in ileocaecal or mesenteric lymph nodes is the best diagnostic test either at postmortem or by biopsy.
- Faecal culture – probably the next most reliable antemortem test but requires 8–12 weeks and will not detect less than 100 organisms/g thereby missing some carrier animals.
- Agar gel immunodiffusion test – correlates reasonably well with faecal culture; useful for identifying profuse excretors.
- Complement fixation tests – inaccurate; false positives and false negatives occur.
- Intradermal tests – not recommended, false negatives occur.

Postmortem findings

- Emaciation; absence of abdominal fat.
- Mesenteric lymph nodes generally enlarged and oedematous in later stages with foci of caseation.
- Slight thickening and corrugation of the ileal mucosa and possibly of the mucosa of the caecum and proximal colon.
- Even in the absence of gross lesions sections from the mesenteric lymph nodes, distal ileum and ileocaceal valve should be submitted for histological examination.

Treatment

- None.

Control

- Snatch kids at birth (see CAE control) and raise in isolation from the rest of the herd.
- Routine faecal cultures from goats in an infected herd – cull any positive animals and any offspring which have not been snatched.
- Regular cleaning and disinfection of yards and buildings.
- A goat vaccine is available in Norway; in the UK, a bovine vaccine has been used in problem herds.

Liver disease

See also Chapter 14.

Chronic fascioliasis

The liver fluke *Fasciola hepatica* can cause acute, subacute or
chronic disease, according to the numbers and stage of
development of the parasite in the liver. Acute fascioliasis
occurs when large numbers of immature fluke cause massive
destruction of liver tissue resulting in liver failure and
haemorrhage. Subacute fascioliasis occurs when large numbers
of fluke are ingested over a longer period, so that as well as
immature fluke in the liver parenchyma, there are adult fluke in
the major bile ducts. Chronic fascioliasis is the result of liver
damage caused by migrating fluke and blood loss caused by
adult flukes in the bile ducts. The browsing habits of goats mean
that large numbers of infective metacercariae are unlikely to be
ingested over a short period so that although acute and subacute
disease does occur, the chronic form is more common. There is
no immunity to reinfection with *F. hepatica*.

Diagnosis

• Clinical signs, faecal egg counts and postmortem.

Treatment

• Treat the whole herd/flock.
   (1) Chronic fascioliasis – oxyclozanide 15 mg/kg (Levafas,
       Norbrook Laboratories; Zanil, Coopers Pitman-Moore)
       only drug licensed for use in goats; no milk witholding
       time.
       Albendazole (Valbazen, Norden laboratories) at 7.5 mg/kg
       is effective against adult fluke as well as gastrointestinal
       worms and tapeworms but is not licensed for use in goats.
   (2) Acute and subacute fascioliasis – oxyclozanide 45 mg/kg.
       Other drugs, e.g. diamphenethide (Corban, Coopers
       Pitman-Moore) or triclabendazole (Fasinex, Ciba Geigy)
       are more effective against immature fluke but are not
       licensed for use in goats or for use in milk producing
       animals.

Control

• Reduce availability of snail populations.
   (1) drainage
   (2) fencing
   (3) molluscicides.

Table 8.1 Fascioliasis

Type		Clinical signs	Fluke number	Eggs/g faeces	Clinical pathology	Postmortem
Chronic	January to April	Progressive weight loss Anaemia Oedema, ascites	250+ (adults)	100+	Hypochromic macrocytic anaemia Eosinophilia, hypoalbuminaemia AST (other liver enzymes normal)	Hepatic fibrosis Hyperplastic cholangitis
Acute	October to January	Sudden death Abdominal pain Dyspnoea, ascites	1000+ (mainly immature)	0	Nomochromic normocytic anaemia Eosinophilia, hypoalbuminaemia AST, GGT, SDH, GDH	Liver enlarged and haemorrhagic Tracts of migrating fluke Fibrinous peritonitis
Subacute	October to January	Rapid weight loss Anaemia Submandibular oedema Ascites	500–1500 (adults + immature)	<100	Hypochromic macrocytic anaemia Eosinophilia, hypoalbuminaemia	As acute + bile ducts distended by adult fluke

- Prophylactic use of fluke anthelmintics – in non-lactating animals use of diamphenethide or triclabendazole in March and May will prevent pasture contamination with fluke eggs.

MAFF forecasts based on the temperature and rainfall in the spring and early summer annually, so that specific control measures can be varied according to the predicted incidence of disease.

Abscess

Abscesses may arise:

- In kids following a navel infection.
- Following a septicaemia.
- In caseous lymphadenitis.

Tumour

Primary tumours of the liver are rare, occasional secondary tumours occur.

Ragwort poisoning

See Chapter 20.

Visceral cysticercosis

Cystercus tenuicollis is the metacestode of the carnivore tapeworm *Taenia hydatigena*. After ingestion, migrating cysts pass through the liver. Infection with small numbers is inapparent, but large numbers of cysts will cause widespread damage to the liver parenchyma (hepatitis cysticercosa) and result in depression, anorexia, pyrexia, weight loss, abdominal discomfort and occasionally death in kids. Acute disease is rarely seen in animals over 6 months of age.

The migrating cysts may lead to infection with *Clostridium oedematiens* type B ('Black Disease') (see Chapter 18).

Hydatid disease

Hydatid cysts are the metacestode stage of the carnivore tapeworm *Echinococcus granulosus*. The cysts initially develop in the liver and in high numbers may cause vascular or biliary obstruction in the liver. A local host response may lead to necrosis and infection of the liver. However, clinical disease is uncommon, large numbers of cysts being carried by apparently healthy animals. A proportion of cysts reach the lungs and may produce respiratory signs, particularly if a secondary infection, e.g. Pasteurellosis, occurs.

Public Health considerations

- Hydatid cysts can also infect man. Although the goat is not a direct source of human infection, an infected animal would indicate environmental contamination and control of tape-worm infection in dogs should be instigated.

Aflatoxicosis

Goats are relatively resistant to aflatoxins – the clinical signs are similar to those caused by other hepatotoxins such as pyrrolizidone alkaloids, e.g. ragwort.

Interference with rumen/intestinal mobility

- Chronic rumen impaction (see Chapter 14).
- Ascites
    fascioliasis (qv)
    passive congestion of the liver.
- Ruminoreticular ulceration.
- Adhesions following surgery (e.g. caesarian section).
- Tumour – carcinomas (rare, older goats).
- Cestode infection (see Chapter 13)?; if present in sufficient numbers could occlude intestinal lumen otherwise unlikely to cause weight loss.
- Left-sided displacement of the abomasum – see Chapter 14 and Periparturient toxaemia.

Presence of chronic disorders

Recurrent bouts of pyrexia, toxaemia and lethargy or painful conditions will lead to progressive weight loss.

- Chronic pneumonia
    pasteurella
    CAE
    lungworm infection
    viruses
    (mycoplasma)
    (caseous lymphadenitis).

- Chronic peritonitis.
- Chronic enteritis
  salmonella
  chronic enterotoxaemia?
- Chronic mastitis (see Chapter 12).
- Metritis.
- Tuberculosis.
  rare
  notifiable

Aetiology

- Goats generally infected with *Mycobacterium bovis* but are also susceptible to infection with *M. tuberculosis* and *M. avium*.

Transmission

- Infection can occur by inhalation or ingestion.

Clinical signs

- Goats may have extensive lesions without obvious clinical signs.
- Occurs as a disseminated disease involving the thorax (mediastinal lymph nodes, lungs, pleura) and abdomen (peritoneum, liver, spleen, mesenteric lymph nodes); occasionally superficial lymph nodes are enlarged and palpable.
- Chronic weight loss ± diarrhoea.
- Chronic cough due to bronchopneumonia.
- Skin lesions occassionally present – fistulae, ulcers and nodules.

Postmortem findings

- Tuberculosis granulomas in one or more lymph nodes.
- Caseous tubercles in lung, liver or spleen.

Diagnosis

- Single intradermal or comparative intradermal test as for cattle.
- False positives and false negatives occur.

Public health considerations

- *M. bovis* can be excreted in milk, faeces, urine, vaginal discharges, expired air and discharges from skin lesions or lymph nodes.

Pruritic conditions

- Lice (see Chapter 10) – often present in large numbers in chronically wasted goats either.
  (1) as secondary opportunists when a goat is in poor condition for any other cause or
  (2) very occasionally as a primary cause of weight loss through pruritis and anaemia when there is a heavy infestation.
- Sarcoptic mange (see Chapter 10).
- Scrapie (see Chapter 11).

Further reading

General

Buchan, G. A. G. (1988) The wasting goat. *Goat Vet. Soc. J.*, **10** (2), 58–63

East, N. E. (1982) Chronic weight loss in adult dairy goats. *Comp. Cont. Ed. Pract. Vet*, **4** (10), S419–S424

Sherman, D. M. (1983) Unexplained weight loss in sheep and goats. *Vet. Clin. North Amer.: Large Animal Practice*, **5** (3), November 1983, 571–590

Nutrition

Oldham, J. D. and Mowlem, A. (1981) Feeding goats for milk producton. *Goat Vet. Soc. J.*, **2** (1), 13–19

Randall, E. M. (1985) Nutrition in late pregnancy and early lactation. *Goat Vet. Soc. J.*, **6** (2), 51–55

Randall, E. M. (1988) Caprine nutrition. *Goat Vet. Soc. J.*, **10** (1), 28–33

Suttle, N. F. (1989) Predicting risks of mineral disorders in goats. *Goat Vet. Soc. J.*, **10** (1), 19–27

Webster, A. J. F. (1988) Goat nutrition. *Goat Vet. Soc. J.*, **10** (1), 46–49

Johne's disease

Baxendell, S. A. (1984) Johne's disease in goats. *Proc. Univ. Sydney Post Grad. Comm. Vet. Sci.*, **73**, 508–510

Saxegaard, F. and Fodstad, F. H. (1985) Control of paratuberculosis in goats by vaccination. *Vet. Rec.*, **116**, 439–441

Thomas, G. W. (1983) Paratuberculosis in a large goat herd. *Vet. Rec.*, **113**, 464–466

Liver fluke

Taylor, M. (1987) Liverfluke treatment. *In Practice*, September 1987, 163–166

Periparturient toxaemia

Andrews, A. M. (1985) Some metabolic conditions in the doe. *Goat. Vet. Soc. J.*, **6**, 70–72

Baxendell, S. A. (1984) Pregnancy toxaemia. *Proc. Univ. Sydney Post. Grad. Comm. Vet. Sci.*, **73**, 548–556

Merrall, M. (1985) Nutritional and metabolic diseases. *In Proc. Course in Goat Husbandry and Medicine, Massey University,* November 1985, 126–151

Pinsent, J. and Cottom, D. S. (1987) Metabolic diseases of goats. *Goat Vet. Soc. J.,* **8** (1), 40–42

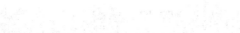

9 External swellings

Throat swellings

- Thymus enlargement
  (a) thymic hyperplasia/non-regression of the thymus
  (b) thymoma
  (c) fat in the thymus.
- Wattle cysts.
- Salivary cysts.
- Thyroid enlargement
  (a) goitre
  (b) iodine excess.
- Tumours
    lymphosarcoma
    malignant melanoma.

Head and neck swellings

- Abscess.
- Vaccination reaction.
- Tooth root abscesses.
- Bottle jaw.
- Impacted cud.
- 'Big head'.
- Tumours.
- Orf.
- Herpes virus.
- Mycotic dermatitis (Dermotophilosis).
- Ringworm.
- Actinomycosis.

Body swellings

- Abscess.
- Haematoma/seroma.
- Tumour.
- Hernia.
- Prolapse.
- Umbilical abscess.
- Ectopic mammary tissue.
- Ticks.
- Keds.
- Cyst.
- (Warble flies.)

Legs

- Orf.
- Chorioptic mange.
- Mycotic dermatitis (strawberry footrot).

Throat swellings

The differential diagnosis for throat swellings should include the following.

Thymus enlargement

Thymic hyperplasia/non-regression of the thymus

A common condition in kids resulting in soft swellings in the ventral neck region. Probably a normal developmental occurrence – often confused by owners with 'goitre' (qv).

Thymoma

A relatively common tumour in adult goats, operable if relatively small but may extend into the chest cavity, preventing swallowing and regurgitation by pressure on the oesophagus at the thoracic inlet or producing respiratory or cardiac dysfunction. Thymic tumours may form part of a multicentric lymphosarcoma complex.

Fat in the thymus

Wattle cysts

An inherited fault occurring particularly in British Alpine and Anglo Nubian goats, resulting in a swelling at the base of one or both wattles varying from peasize to several centimetres diameter. Surgical removal may be requested if the cyst is unsightly, particularly in show goats.

Diagnosis

- The position of the cyst is diagnostic.
- Histopathology is confirmatory revealing walls of stratified squamous epithelium with mature hair follicles.

Salivary cysts

A relatively common condition, particularly in Anglo Nubians. The cyst arises from damage to the submandibular or parotid salivary glands or their ducts with formation of a mucocoele containing saliva.

Treatment

- Surgical removal if indicated.

Thyroid enlargement

Thyroid enlargement presents as swellings either side of the trachea.

Goitre (see Chapter 5)

Owners commonly associate *any* throat swelling with 'goitre', treat with iodine and risk iodine overdose. Genuine goitre is rare.

Iodine excess (see Chapter 5)

Iodine overdosage will in itself produce enlarged thyroid glands.

Tumours

Lymphosarcoma

Multicentric lymphosarcomas usually involve generalized enlargement of the lymph nodes, particularly in the face and shoulder region with lesions in the spleen, liver, kidney or intestines. Occasionally the disease is more localized, with the jaw region a predilection site.

Malignant melanoma

Malignant melanomas (qv) often spread rapidly via the lymphatic system to involve the lymph nodes of the neck.

Other swellings around the head and neck

Abscess

- Abscessation or cellulitis may arise occasionally as the result of tissue penetration by a number of different bacteria.

- An injection abscess may arise at the site of vaccination or other injection because of faulty injection techniques (but most swellings produced by vaccination are sterile – see below).
- Caseous lymphadenitis – a chronic bacterial infection caused by *Corynebacterium pseudotuberculosis* and characterized by the swelling of lymph nodes in various parts of the body. The disease has recently been reported in the UK and is common worldwide. The abscesses are particularly common in the head and neck region, prescapular lymph nodes and prefemoral and superficial inguinal lymph nodes.

Vaccination reaction

Sterile swellings commonly occur as a reaction to the clostridial vaccine adjuvant (particularly if oil-based) and may range in size from small nodules to several centimetres in diameter. Some animals seem particularly sensitive to any clostridial vaccine, others will react to only one particular product. In show animals vaccination on the sternum may be preferable to the neck or scapular regions.

Tooth root abscess

Tooth root abscesses present as a lump on the upper or lower jaw, often closely associated with the bone, sometimes with an associated cellulitis.

An abscess of the lower jaw may track to the outside on the mandible; an abscess of the upper jaw may discharge into the mouth or sinuses of the skull.

Bottle jaw

'Bottle jaw' is a soft fluid-filled swelling under the jaw as a result of anaemia, particularly haemonchosis. Other signs of anaemia will also be present.

Impacted cud

Dental abnormalities, such as worn or poorly aligned molars in older goats may result in retention and impaction of cud in the mouth producing swollen cheeks.

'Big head'

Clostridial infections (*C.novyi or C.oedematiens*) in bucks which have been fighting produce a swollen head as part of an acute illness association with lethargy, anorexia and pyrexia.

Tumours

The incidence of skin tumours is very low in the UK. The major tumours – papillomas, squamous cell carcinomas and malignant melanomas – occur most commonly in white dairy or Angora goats with non-pigmented skin exposed to strong sunlight, so the incidence is likely to remain low unless the greenhouse effect produces a dramatic climate change!

Cutaneous papillomas

Papillomatosis is caused by a virus of the papovirus group. Three types of papillomas have been described in the goat.

- Mammary.
- Cutaneous.
- Genital.

Cutaneous papillomas occur particularly on the head, neck and thoracic limb and are flat, circumscribed with a crusty surface and ringwormlike appearance.

Generally a spontaneous resolution occurs in a few months. Occasionally surgical removal or the use of autogenous vaccines is indicated.

Squamous cell carcinomas

Squamous cell carcinomas occur particularly perianally, around the vulva and udder and on the eyelid and nictitating membrane in areas of non-pigmented skin in response to stimulation by ultraviolet irridation. In the early stages the tumours appear as thickened areas of skin, enlarging rapidly and becoming ulcerated and often coalescing to form large masses.

Malignant melanoma

Malignant melanomas commonly occur on the head and ears, occasionally the vulva or perianally, arising as small firm nodules from black pigmented areas and enlarging rapidly to form a black mass. Rapid spread via the lymphatic system may occur to involve the regional lymph nodes. Some melanomas may be unpigmented and resemble squamous cell carcinomas.

Other tumours

Fibromas and fibrosarcomas have occasionally been reported from the head region of goats.

Orf (contagious ecthyma; contagious pustular dermatitis)

A poxvirus infection causing pustules and then crusty, scabby lesions on the commissures of the lips, gums, nostrils, buccal mucosa and occasionally the udder, feet or tail. Unlike papillomas which are firmly attached to the skin, orf scabs can be picked off revealing inflamed, granulating areas.

Debilitation and even death may occur if painful lesions prevent feeding. Local secondary bacterial infections may occur.

Diagnosis

- The virus can be demonstrated in fresh scabs by electron microscopy. Submit scabs from fresh lesions to the laboratory in a screwtopped container.

Treatment

- Secondary bacterial infection can be controlled with antibiotic sprays.

Prevention

- In infected herds vaccination (Scabivax, Coopers Pitman-Moore) can be considered; live virus will be shed for 3–4 weeks. Vaccinate in the tail fold or inside the ear.

Public health considerations

- Orf causes localized lesions on hands or forearms.

Herpes virus

Herpes viruses have been identified as causing wartlike lesions on the eyelid and proliferative lesions around the mouth and hard palate as well as vulvovaginitis, abortion, ulcerative enteritis and pneumonia (? presence in UK).

Diagnosis

- Culture of virus; serology.

Mycotic dermatitis (Dermatophilosis)

See Chapter 6.

Ringworm

See Chapter 10.

Actinomycosis ('lumpy jaw')

Occurs rarely in goats, mimicking the bovine disease and producing hard painful swellings on the mandible and maxilla.

Diagnosis

• Direct smears, culture in anaerobic conditions or biopsy show gram-positive filamentous organism *Actimomyces bovis.*

Treatment

• Intramuscular/local antibiotics; surgical excision and drainage.

Body swellings

(1) Abscess
(2) Haematoma/seroma
(3) Tumour – reported tumours include squamous cell carcinoma, melanoma, lymphosarcoma, papilloma, haemangioma and histiocytoma.
(4) Hernia
    umbilical
    scrotal
    perineal
    ventral
(5) Prolapse
    rectal (see Chapter 4)
    vaginal (see Chapter 4)
(6) Umbilical abscess – associated with joint ill.
(7) Ectopic mammary tissue – may result in a bilateral enlargement of the vulva lips in late pregnancy.
(8) Ticks – the sheep tick *Ixodes ricinus* is sometimes found on goats grazing sheep pastures. The hedgehog tick, *I.hexagonus* is also occasionally identified.

(9) Keds – the sheep ked, *Melophagus ovinus*, occasionally infects goats.
(10) Coenurus cyst of *Taenia multiceps* can occur as a sub-cutaneous cyst.
(11) Warble flies – typical swellings under the skin on the back have been reported, although not from the UK.

Legs

(1) Orf – see 'Head and neck swellings'.
(2) Chorioptic mange – see Chapter 10.
(3) Strawberry footrot (mycotic dermatitis) – see Chapter 10.

Further reading

Brown, C. C. and Olander, H. J. (1987) Caseous lymphadenitis of goats and sheep, a review. *Vet. Bull.*, **57** (1), 1–12

Brown, P. J. *et al.* (1989) Developmental cysts in the upper neck of Anglo-Nubian goats. *Vet. Rec.*, **125**, 256–258

Fubini, S. L. and Campbell, S. G. (1983) External lumps on sheep and goats. *Vet. Clin. North Amer.: Large Animal Practice*, **5** (3), Nov. 1983, 457–476

Gilmour, N. J. L. (1990) Caseous lymphadenitis: a cause for concern. *Vet. Rec.*, **126**, 566

Pritchard. G. C. (1988) Throat swellings in goats. *GVS J.*, **10** (1)

Rijnberk, A. *et al.* (1977) Congenital defect in iodothyronine synthesis, clinical aspects of iodine metabolism in goats with congenital goitre and hypothyroidism. *Br. Vet. J.*, **133**, 495–503

Williams, C. S. F. (1980) Differential diagnosis of caseous lymphadenitis in the goat. *VMSAC*, **75**, 1165

10 Skin disease

Skin disease causing pruritis

- Lice.
- Sarcoptic mange.
- Fly worry.
- Harvest mites.
- Forage mites.
- Scrapie .
- Psoroptic mange.
- Strongyloides papillosus.
- Onchocerca.
- Pemphigus foliaceous.
- Photosensitization.

Non-pruritic skin disease

- Chorioptic mange.
- Demodectic mange.
- Staphylococcal dermatitis.
- Orf.
- Zinc deficiency.
- Urine scald.
- Alopecia/hyperkeratosis in older bucks.
- Trauma.
- Labial dermatitis in kids.
- Ringworm.
- Pygmy goat syndrome.
- Golden Guernsey goat syndrome.
- Mycotic dermatitis.
- Iodine deficiency.
- Selenium/vitamin E deficiency.

Initial assessment

The preliminary history should consider:

- Clinical signs observed by owner and how long present.
- Individual or herd problem.
- Contact with goats and other animals.
- General health of affected goat and of herd.
- Response to any treatment given.
- Management (feeding, worming etc.).

General clinical examination

The goat should be carefully examined:

- For signs of intercurrent disease, e.g. helminthiasis.
- To assess its behaviour (rubbing, nibbling, pruritis etc.); study the goat, preferably in its own surroundings.
- To assess the general conditon of the animal – weight etc.; evidence of malnutrition. Malnourished goats will have dry scaly skin often with a heavy lice burden.

Examination of skin

- Head/neck – particularly periorbital area and pinnae; mouth and mucocutaneous junction of lips.
- Thorax/abdomen – particularly axillae, udder and inguinal regions.
- Perineal region.
- Legs and feet.

Record

- Distribution of lesions (use sketches if indicated).
- Type and size of lesions.
- Quality of skin – colour, elasticity, odour, temperature.
- Response of animal to palpation of lesions.
- Hair loss or damage to follicles.
- Skin secretions.
- Self-inflicted damage.

Laboratory tests

(1) *Hair sample* – pluck with tweezers from edge of active lesion.
   (i) Direct microscopy – identification of ringworm.

NB Wood's lamp normally *negative* in goats with ringworm.

   (ii) Culture
        fungal media (ringworm)
        blood agar (*Dermatophilus congolensis*).
(2) *Skin swab* – from active lesion near scaly or scabby area.
   - Culture on blood agar – *Staph.aureus* in pure culture is generally significant, but may be a secondary infection.

(3) Impression smear – of pus under a crust.
- Stain with Dip Quick, Giemsa or new methylene blue
- Useful for *Dermatophilus congolensis* and candidiasis.

(4) Skin scrapings – essential for diagnosis of some manges. Scraping taken from each of a number of active lesions, collected and covered with potassium hydroxide before being warmed in a waterbath overnight.
- Sarcoptic mange – mites difficult to find; diagnosis difficult from scrape.
- Demodectic mange – many mites found when nodule expressed
- Chorioptic and psoroptic mange – mites easily found in scrapes from legs and ears respectively.

(5) Skin biopsy – whole thickness skin strips taken under local anaesthesia; preferably from normal, marginal and abnormal areas; fix in formol saline.

(6) Electron microscopy – useful in diagnosis of orf; scabs fixed in buffered gluteraldehyde.

(7) Blood sample
- Anaemia (lice infestation etc.).
- Neutrophilia (bacterial infection).
- Eosinophilia (allergic, parasitic infestation).

Pruritic skin disease

Lice

The biting louse *Damalinia caprae* and the blood sucking louse *Linognathus stenopsis* affect goats, producing pruritus and hair loss particularly on the head, neck and back. Lice are very common and in articomplicate the problem by producing anaemia (qv). The damage to fleece can cause financial loss in Angora goats.

Diagnosis

Lice are visible to the naked eye.

Sarcoptic mange

Relatively common disease affecting goats of all ages. Transmitted primarily by direct contact but also by indirect contact such as milking, handling etc.

Clinical signs

- Lesions start around the eyes and ears with erythema and small nodules, progressing to hair loss, thickening and wrinkling of the skin, in response to intense pruritus and scratching over the head, neck and body. Secondary infection with *Staph. aureus* is common.
- Affected goats often lose condition and the milk yield falls because of the intensity of the irritation.

Diagnosis

- Demonstration of the mite, *Sarcoptes scabiei*, in deep skin scrapings may be extremely difficult as very few mites can be found even with severe lesions; skin biopsy may demonstrate mites.

Fly worry

Biting flies are particularly worrying to housed goats in the summer producing quite severe lesions resembling superficially staphylococcal dermatitis on the udder but generally more pruritic. Topical creams and washes will ease the lesions. Control of flies in the goat house will help prevent the problem, e.g. Golden Malrin (Sanoffi).

Myiasis (blowfly strike) is much less common than in sheep but may occur around the head following fights, in wounds in soiled areas around the tail, breech and penis or the feet of animals with footrot/scald.

Other external parasites

Harvest mites, forage mites, *Cheyletiella*, fleas and poultry mites (*Dermanyssus gallinae*) are occasionally reported to cause pruritic skin disease in goats.

Scrapie (see Chapter 11)

Scrapie causes pruritis and self-mutilation but is not as pruritic in goats as sheep.

Psoroptic mange

Psoroptes cuniculi parasitizes the ear, generally without clinical signs occasionally producing head shaking and scratching. Scaly

Table 10.1 External parasites

	Causal agent	Incidence	Distribution of lesions	Lesions	Pruritus	Diagnosis	Treatment
Lice	*Damalinia caprae* (biting) *Linognathus stenopsis* (sucking)	+++	Head, neck, back	Hair loss Broken hairs Motheaten coat	++	Naked eye	Organophosphorus dips γBHC Bromocyclen Pyrethroid pour ons
Chorioptic mange	*Chorioptes*	+++	Lower posterior limb Occ. ventral abdomen, sternum	Crusting Erythema	−	Skin scraping	γBHC Bromocyclen Ivomectin
Demodectic mange	*Demodex caprae*	++	Head, neck, body	Hard nodules with yellow caseous material	−	Microscopy on expressed material skin biopsy	Rotenone
Pustular dermatitis	*Staphylococcus aureus*	+++	Udder, teats* ventral abdomen groin, body	Pustular scabs Dry scaly coat	−	Culture[+]	Local/parenteral antibiotics or udder washes

Sarcoptic mange	*Sarcoptes scabiei*	+	Head, ears, body	Alopecia, crusting Self-inflicted damage Lymph nodes Weight loss	+++	Skin biopsy (skin scraping)	Ivomectin, γBHC
Ringworm	*Trichophyton verrucosium* *Microsporum canis* *Trichophyton mentagraphytes*	Rare	Head, body	Raised, circular crusty	–	Microscopy culture	Griseofulvin in feed Topical prep.
Psoroptic mange	*Psoroptes cuniculi*	Rare	Ear (head, body)	Head shaking	++	Skin scraping	γBHC
Harvest mites		Rare	Legs, face, lower body	Exudative patches	++	Naked eye	γBHC

* see Udder disease
† NB *Staph.aureus* is often a secondary invader in other skin conditions, e.g. mange

Table 10.2 Treatment of external parasites

		Lice	Chorioptic mange	Sarcoptic mange	Demodectic mange	Psoroptic mange	Ticks/keds	Milk withholding time	Meat withholding time
γBHC	Univet louse powder*	+					+	NS	NS
	Quellada	+		+			+	NS	NS
	Auroid GAC ear drops					+		–	–
Lindane	Coopers louse powder	+					+	Not for lactating animals	NS
Cypemethrin	Ovipor*	+					+	6 hours	7 days
	Parasol*	+					+	6 hours	7 days
Deltamethrin	Spoton	+					+	Nil for cattle/sheep	3 days (sheep/cattle)
Coumaphos	Asuntol powder	+					+	Treat after milking (cattle)	NS
	Asuntol*	+					+	Treat after milking	NS

Bromocyclen	Alugan dusting powder	+			+	NS	NS
	Alugan aerosol spray	+	+		+	NS	NS
	Alugan conc. powder	+	+		+	NS	NS
Ivermectin	Ivomec injection	±	?†	+	+	28 days (cattle)	21 days (cattle)
Rotenone	Head to tail demodectic mange dressing			+		NS	NS

NS – not stated

* Product licensed for use in goats

† Care should be taken in animals producing milk or meat for human consumption when products are not licensed for use in goats. Ivermectin will kill blood sucking lice but not biting or non-burrowing mites. Repeat injections will sometimes kill chorioptic mites. Asuntol is the only dip licensed for use in goats in the UK at present, but dipping in organophosphorus insecticides such as diazinon or propetamphos will control external parasites.

lesions may be found on the inside of the pinnae and occasionally on the head, neck or body. Kids are infected by their dams and may show clinical signs by 3 weeks of age. Severe vestibular disease and facial nerve paralysis may occur if the tympanic membrane ruptures.

Diagnosis

- Identification of mite; larger than *Chorioptes* with long jointed pedicel and trumpet shaped suckers.

Strongyloidiasis

A localized dermatitis can occur as part of the immune response to the larvae of *Strongyloides papillosus*. Affects lower limbs causing pruritus with stamping and nibbling.

Onchocerca

Onchocerca produces fine skin nodules particularly in the neck and shoulder region with mild pruritus.

Autoimmune skin disease

Pemphigus foliaceous has been diagnosed in goats showing crusty pruritic lesions on the skin in the perineal and scrotal regions and on the ventral abdomen. Diagnosis confirmed by skin biopsy.

Photosensitization

Causes pruritus, erythema, oedema and swelling of the skin, with blistering and scab formation.

(1) Primary – due to ingestion of St John's wort (*Hypericum perforatom*) or buckwheat (*Fagopyrum esculentum*).
(2) Secondary – in animals with hepatic dysfunction due to accumulation of phylloerythrin, a breakdown derivative of chlorophyll. Any liver damage affecting bile excretion may be implicated – liver disease, hepatotoxic drugs, chemicals, mycotoxins or plant toxins, (e.g. bog asphodel (*Northecium ossifragum*)).

Treatment

- Prevent access to any photosensitizing plant, protect from sunlight, symptomatic and supportive therapy.

Non-pruritic skin disease

Chorioptic mange

Very common infection of goats in the UK, particularly in housed goats in the winter but occurring throughout the year. Legs should always be checked for chorioptic mange during routine foot trimming.

Clinical signs

- White/brown scabby lesions generally at the back of the pasterns but occasionally extending as far as the knee or hock in severe infection. Very occasionally lesions may be found on the ventral abdomen, sternum or even upper body. Lesions may be complicated with a *Staph. aureus* infection.

Diagnosis

- Microscopical identification of non-burrowing mite *Chorioptes caprae*.
  Mites generally easily found; short pedicel with flask shaped suckers on legs.

Demodectic Mange (*Demodex caprae*)

Relatively common, particularly in British Alpine goats. Goatlings most commonly show clinical disease following infection as a kid. Usually an individual rather than a herd problem.

Clinical signs

- Small nodules (generally about 1–2 cm) in the skin of the head, neck and body due to multiplication of the mite in individual sebaceous glands. Yellow caseous material, containing numerous mites, can be expressed from the nodules.

Diagnosis

- Microscopical identification of mites in caseous material from nodules. Very easy to find in smears. Cigar shaped body with bluntly pointed abdomen.

Staphylococcal dermatitis (pustular dermatitis)

Staph. aureus infection is very common, causing pustules of variable size up to 4 cm especially on the udder, teats and groin but also ventral abdomen and occasionally any part of the body. First kidders are particularly affected soon after parturition. Pustules are easily broken and spread, healing as a scabby or impetigo-like lesion and infection may be spread between goats at milking by hands, cloths or milking dusters. The lesions are generally non-painful and milk yield is not affected.

The disease is colloquially known as 'goat pox' but true 'goat pox' caused by capripoxvirus does not occur in the UK.

NB Staph. aureus is a common secondary invader of other skin lesions.

Orf

See 'External swellings' (Chapter 9).

Zinc deficiency

Probably more common than generally recognized. Diets should generally be adequate in zinc, but (1) an excess of copper will interfere with zinc uptake as will a high calcium intake (e.g. lucerne); (2) Individual goats may not absorb adequate amounts; (3) some male goats may have higher requirements.

Clinical signs

- Hair loss; hyperkeratosis and parakeratosis with thickened, wrinkled skin particularly hind limbs, scrotum, neck and head.
- Hair loss on the ears of Anglo Nubian kids has also responded emperically to zinc supplements.

NB Zinc deficiency may also result in infertility with low conception rates.

Laboratory tests

- Zinc blood levels can be estimated using a sample taken into a sodium citrate vacutainer, but correlation between serum and dietary zinc levels may be poor.

Treatment

- Zinc sulphate drench 1% or zinc sulphate tablets, 250 mg to 1 g daily orally for 2–4 weeks.

Urine scald

Male goats urinate on themselves during the breeding season, particularly down the back of the forelegs, face and beard and this will result in staining, hair loss and possibly scalding of the skin.

Similarly staining will occur on goats that are recumbent or housed in dirty conditions.

Alopecia/skin thickening in older male goats

Older male goats (particularly British Toggenburg and British Alpine) commonly have thickened scaley skin especially over the head and back, possibly due in part to urine scald, nutritional deficiency during the breeding season (zinc related?) and as a response to rubbing, although the exact aetiology is unknown.

Treatment with baby oils or olive oil thinned with surgical spirit has been suggested as suitable for removing excess scaling to allow new hair to grow, following thorough shampooing. Zinc sulphate supplements should also be considered.

Trauma

Labial dermatitis in artificially reared kids

Kids reared artificially may develop erythema and hair loss around the face and mouth due to wetting. Occasionally a secondary infection with *Staph. aureus* occurs (see Pustular dermatitis). Needs distinguishing from the early stages of Orf (see Chapter 9) and from Dermatophilosis (see Chapter 6).

Ringworm

Ringworm is an uncommon infection acquired from other hosts. *Trichophyton verrucosum* from cattle is seen most frequently, occasionally *T.mentagrophytes* from rodents and *Microsporum canis* from dogs or cats.

Lesions are initially circular, crusty and raised, later irregular in shape, often occurring on the head, ears and neck.

Diagnosis

- Microscopy and culture.
- Trichophyton species do *not* fluoresce under a Wood's lamp.

Treatment

- Griseofulvin in food for 7 days or local fungicides.

Pygmy goat syndrome

Certain families of pygmy goats develop non-pruritic crusty lesions around the eyes, ears, nose and head and in the axilla, groin and perineal region. Aetiology unknown.

Golden Guernsey goat syndrome ('sticky kid')

An hereditary disease caused by an autosomal recessive gene. Affected kids are born with sticky, greasy matted coats which remain abnormal throughout life.

Mycotic dermatitis (dermatophilosis)

See Chapter 6.

Iodine deficiency

See Chapter 5.
   May result in weak kids born with thin sparse hair coat as part of a syndrome of abortion, weak kids and still births. Older goats may show poor growth rate and dry scabby skin as a result of general malnutrition.

Selenium/vitamin E deficiency

May produce a dry coat and dandruff.

Skin disease presenting as swellings (qv)

(1) Neoplasia
       papillomatosis
       melanoma
       squamous cell carcinoma
       haemangioma
(2) Orf
(3) Ticks – *I.ricinus* (sheeptick), *I.hexagonus* (hedgehog tick).
       Keds – *Melophagus ovinus* (sheep ked).
(4) Abscess

Further reading

Jackson, P. (1982) Skin disease in goats. *Goat Vet. Soc. J.*, **3** (1), 7–11
Jackson, P. (1986) Skin diseases in goats. *In Practice*, January 1986, 5–10
Jackson, P., Richards, H. W. and Lloyds (1983) Sarcoptic mange in goats. *Vet. Rec.*, **112**, 330
Scott, D. W., Smith, M. C. and Manning, T. O. (1984) Caprine dermatology. Part I. *Comp. Cont. Ed. Pract. Vet.*, **6** (4), S190–S211
Scott, D. W., Smith, M. C. and Manning, T. O. (1984) Caprine dermatology. Part II. *Comp. Cont. Ed. Pract. Vet.*, **6** (8), S473–S485
Smith, M. C. (1981) Caprine dermatologic problems: a review. *JAVMA*, **178**, 724
Smith, M. C. (1983) Dermatologic diseases of goats. *Vet. Clin. North Amer.: Large Animal Practice*, **5** (3), Nov. 1983, 449–456
Walton, G. S. (198) Skin lesions and goats. *Goat Vet. Soc. J.*, **1** (2), 15–16
Wright, A. I. (1989) Dermatology. *Goat Vet. Soc. J.*, **10** (2), 64–66

11 Nervous diseases

Neonatal kids

- Congenital infections.
- Hypoglycaemia.
- Birth trauma.
- Enzootic ataxia (swayback).

Kids up to one month

- Spinal abscess.
- Trauma.
- Congenital vertebral lesions.
- Tick pyaemia.
- Bacterial meningitis.
- Focal symmetrical encephalomalacia (enterotoxaemia).
- Tetanus.
- Disbudding meningoencephalitis.
- Louping ill.

2–7 months

- Trauma.
- Delayed swayback.
- Spinal abscess.
- Coccidiosis.
- CAE (viral leucoencephalitis).

7 months–adult

Infectious disease

- Listeriosis.
- Scrapie.
- Louping.
- Tetanus.
- CAE.
- Pseudorabies (Aujesky's disease).
- Rabies.

Metabolic disease

- Cerebrocortical necrosis (CCN, polioencephalomalacia).
- Hypocalcaemia (milk fever).
- Hypomagnesaemia (grass tetany).
- Transit tetany.
- Periparturient toxaemia.

Space-occupying lesions of the brain

- Cerebral abscess.
- Coenuriasis (gid).
- Pituitary abscess syndrome.
- Oestrus ovis.

Space-occupying lesions of the spinal cord

- Spinal meningitis.
- Spinal abscess.
- Vertebral osteomyelitis.
- Tumour.
- Coenuriasis.
- Cerebrospinal nematodiasis.

Trauma

Vestibular disease

- Otitis media/interna.
- Ear mite infection.

Hepatic encephalopathy

Poisonings

- Lead.
- Plant.
- Organophosphates.
- Rafoxanide.
- Urea.

Epilepsy

In addition animals with severe anaemia, liver, kidney, lung or myocardial disease may present with apparent nervous dysfunction.

Initial assessment

The preliminary history should consider:

- Herd/flock or individual problem.
- Age.
- Sex.
- Stage of pregnancy/lactation.
- Diet/dietary changes.

Specific management practices should be discussed.

- Disbudding, castration, dipping.
- Prophylactic therapies – coccidiostats, anthelmintics.
- Feeding/grazing routine.

A careful study of the environment should be made.

- Feed sources – silage, grazing.
- Water sources.
- Fertilizers/weed killers.
- Trace element availability.
- Possible sources of poison.

Clinical examination

- Examine the animal(s) undisturbed in their usual surroundings – bright, alert, responsive or dull and depressed.
- Response to approach – apprehension, trembling etc.
- Head carriage
  hyperaesthesia
  defective vision
  head tilt
  tremors
  head pressing
  lateral deviation
  circling movements.
- Ability to rise – opisthotonus, coma, semicoma.
- Locomotion – move animal slowly at first, then faster. Watch for knuckling, circling, incoordination, ataxia, aimless wandering.
- Physical examination – general examination plus specific features referable to neurological disorders, e.g. drooping of ear or eyelid, facial paralysis, retention of cud, nystagmus, size of pupils.

- Examine eye with ophthalmoscope.
- Specific neurological examination – refer to appropriate text book; techniques applicable to dog or cat can be used in goats.

Cerebrospinal fluid collection

Lumbosacral space

Restrain animal in lateral recumbency with hind legs pulled forward to flex the spine; prepare site surgically and block with local anaesthetic.

Insert 0.9 × 38 mm spinal needle or 0.9 × 38 mm disposable needle into the depression between the last lumbar and first sacrodorsal spinous process; advancing the needle slowly until a slight pop is felt when the dura mater is penetrated. Approximately 1 ml of CSF per 5 kg body weight can be collected.

Atlanto-occipital site

Samples obtained from this site are more likely to represent accurately intracranial lesions but sedation or general anaesthesia is necessary – use lumbosacral space if the animal is too ill to risk sedation.

Prepare site surgically and place animal in lateral recumbency with head at right angles to neck and horizontal to ground. Insert 0.9 × 38 or 63 mm spinal needle or 0.9 × 38 mm disposable needle with the needle pointing towards the lower jaw and advance *slowly* until the dura mater is penetrated.

NB   *Trauma to the brain stem may cause death.*

Laboratory investigation

- Complete blood count.
- Specific tests as indicated.
- Cerebrospinal fluid analysis and culture.

Cerebrospinal fluid analysis and culture

Collect CSF in EDTA tube for cytological examination and plain tube for biochemical analysis and bacteriological culture.

(1) *Colour* – should be clear and colourless.
    Turbidity indicates viral, bacterial, fungal or parasitic infection.

Yellowish discoloration (xanthochromia) indicates presence of blood pigments from trauma or vascular damage.
(2) *Protein level* – normal goats have a level of 0–39 mg/dl; can be measured with urinary reagent strips; > 1+ is abnormal.

Protein levels are increased in infective conditions, may be slightly elevated in traumatic conditions and remain normal in degenerative congenital or toxic conditions.
(3) *Cell counts* – use undiluted fluid in a haemocytometer; allow cells to settle for 5–10 minutes before counting.

Normal goats have counts of 0–4 white cells/µl.

Elevated white cell counts may be found in viral conditions (mononuclear cells), parasitic conditions (neutrophils, occasionally many eosinophils), and bacterial or fungal infections (usually neutrophils; with listeriosis half neutrophils, half mononuclear cells).

Red cells may be found following trauma.
(4) *Glucose levels* – use urinary reagent strip. Normal levels are about 80% the blood glucose level, i.e. about 70 mg/dl.
(5) *Blood content* – use urinary reagent strip.
(6) *Gram stain* of CSF smear following sedimentation.
(7) *Bacterial culture.*

Postmortem examination

- Many neurological disorders are likely to be fatal or even present as sudden death.

Treatment

Specific treatment should be instigated as soon as a diagnosis is made. Until such time general supportive therapy may be indicated:

(1) *Intravenous fluids* (or subcutaneous fluids if handling stresses the goat) in animals which are not drinking or collapsed.
(2) *Anticonvulsants*
  (a) Diazepam (Valium, Roche) – 0.05–0.4 mg/kg i.v. to effect. Repeat as necessary.
  (b) Phenobarbitone (Sagatal, RMB Animal Health) – 0.44 ml/kg i.v. to effect then 0.22 ml/kg every 8 or 12 hours as required.

(3) Anti-inflammatory drugs to control CNS inflammation
  (a) Flunixin meglumine (Finadyne, Schering Plough) – 2 ml/45 kg i.v. or i.m. every 12 or 24 hours for up to 5 days.
  (b) Phenylbutazone – 2–4 mg/kg i.v. or p.o. every 12–24 hours.
  (c) Methylprednisolone (Solu-medrone V, Upjohn) – 10–30 mg/kg i.v. every 4–6 hours for 24–48 hours.

Neonatal kids

See weak kids (Chapter 5).

- Congenital infections.
- Hypoglycaemia.
- Birth trauma.
- Enzootic ataxia (swayback).

Kids up to one month

Kid mentally alert

Spinal abscess

Spinal abscesses and vertebral osteomyelitis occur sporadically in kids generally following a bacteraemia subsequent to a navel infection.

Aetiology

- A number of bacteria including *Staphylococcal* spp., *C.pyogenes*, *Pasteurella* spp. and *Fusobacterium necrophorum* have been implicated.

Clinical signs

- A gradual onset of clinical signs may occur where abscessation results in increasing compression of the spinal cord with signs progressing from slight hind limb ataxia to complete hind limb paralysis and in these cases long-term broad-spectrum antibiotic therapy or more specific therapy based on CSF culture and sensitivity may be satisfactory. In other cases, acute clinical signs, with paraparesis or tetraparesis and pain around the spinal lesion, may occur some time after the original infection when there is sudden collapse of a vertebra and spinal cord compression.

Diagnosis

- Radiography will demonstrate a collapsed vertebra. CSF may appear normal or show increased numbers of neutrophils.

Trauma

In all age groups, trauma to the head or spinal cord may cause neurological signs. Kids are particularly prone to spinal cord and vertebral injuries because of their inquisitive active nature.

Hay nets should be avoided and the spacing on hayracks or gates should be chosen carefully. Trauma can also arise from kicks or bites from other species of animals and from fighting, and neck injuries can also occur in tethered goats.

Pathological vertebral fractures can occur in malnourished animals. Exostosis may develop over incomplete fractures of a vertebral body and subsequently produce neurological signs.

Congenital vertebral lesions

Congenital vertebral lesions can result in compression of the spinal cord with resulting neurological clinical signs, which may not become apparent for several weeks after birth.

Tick pyaemia (enzootic staphylococcal infection)

See Chapter 7.

Kid mentally impaired

Bacterial meningitis

Aetiology

- Generally secondary to septicaemia, with infection from the navel or intestine; enterotoxigenic *E.coli* are generally the causal organisms.

Clinical signs

- Variable neurological signs.
- Lethargy, drowsiness or hyperaesthesia, pyrexia.
- Compulsive wandering; head pressing.
- Nystagmus, apparent blindness.
- Convulsions, coma.
- Death.
- Often history of diarrhoea or diarrhoea present concurrently.

Treatment

- Antibiotic therapy.

  E.coli meningitis is difficult to treat because most bactericidal antibiotics do not penetrate well into the cerebrospinal fluid. Trimethoprim-sulphonamide preparations given intravenously at a level of 16–24 mg of the combined drugs/kg three times daily alone or in combination with gentamicin 3 mg/kg intramuscularly or intravenously (dilute in equal volumes of saline) have been recommended.

  General supportive therapy with fluids, anticonvulsants and anti-inflammatory drugs.

Focal symmetrical encephalomalacia (enterotoxaemia)

Aetiology

- The epsilon toxin produced by *Clostridium perfringens* type D (see Chapter 15) affects the cerebral vasculature producing haemorrhage and oedema.

Clinical signs

- Generally kids, occasionally adult animals.
- Lethargy.
- Head pressing, apparent blindness, trembling.
- Ataxia.
- Opisthotonos, convulsions, coma.
- Death.

NB (1) A similar condition in calves is produced by a labile *coccidial toxin*. It has been suggested that coccidial infections (qv) may be implicated in the condition in kids.

(2) Enterotoxigenic *E.coli* (qv) can also produce similar neurological signs – see bacterial meningitis.

Tetanus

Aetiology

- Gram positive bacillus *Clostridium tetani* produces a neurotoxin responsible for the clinical syndrome.

Epidemiology

Cl.tetani spores enter through wounds following disbudding, castration, shearing, kidding, ear tagging etc. resulting in clinical signs 4–21 days later.

Clinical signs

- Variable neurological signs:
  erect ears, elevated tail, extended neck, rocking horse stance, rigidity and hyperaesthesia on stimulation.
- Prolapsed third eyelid.
- Dysphagia, difficulty in opening mouth.
- Lateral recumbency, death.

Diagnosis

- Clinical signs.
- Isolation and identification of *Cl.tetani*.

Treatment

- Tetanus antitoxin 10 000–15 000 units i.v. twice daily.
- Diazepam (Valium, Roche) 0.05 mg/kg i.v. or acetylpromazine (ACP injection, C-Vet) 0.2 mg/kg i.v. to control muscle spasms.
- Penicillin i.v. and i.m. or ampicillin.
- Supportive therapy – forced feeding, fluids, etc.

Prevention

- Vaccination with a multivalent clostridial vaccine.

Disbudding meningoencephalitis

Prolonged or excessive pressure with a disbudding iron can cause heat necrosis to bone, meninges and brain.

Clinical signs

- Sudden death – sometimes within hours but often several days or even weeks after disbudding.
- Depression, anorexia, pyrexia.

Postmortem findings

- Focal meningoencephalitis.
- Meningeal and superficial cerebrocortical necrosis with infiltration by neutrophils and mononuclear cells.

Louping ill

Aetiology

- Acute encephalomyelitis caused by a flavivirus transmitted by the tick vector *Ixodes ricinus*.

Epidemiology

- Louping ill is transmitted exclusively by the nymph and adult tick. Virus titres which are high enough for tick infection are only obtained in sheep – infection in the goat is thus irrelevant to the maintenance of the viral cycle.
- Strong colostral immunity is imparted to kids so that young animals in endemic areas will be susceptible in their second year of exposure, in contrast to tickborne fever (see Chapter 2) where no colostral protection is conferred, so kids are susceptible during their first season. In endemic areas tickborne fever and louping ill do not simultaneously affect the same animals. However, there is at present widescale movement of goats into endemic areas, so that all ages of goats could be at risk.

Clinical signs

- In adult goats the disease is generally subclinical. Within 24–48 hours of infection a febrile reaction occurs and the temperature may remain elevated for several days before returning to normal. Clinical signs are not usually recognized during this period and neurological signs only develop if the virus gains entry to nervous tissue. In other animals, recovery is rapid and the animals remain immune to subsequent infection. Susceptibility to clinical disease is increased by stress factors such as age, cold, nutrition and transportation and in particular by concurrent infection such as toxoplasmosis and tickborne fever.
- Severe clinical infection can be produced in kids that drink infected milk.
- Lethargy, excessive salivation.
- Intermittent head shaking, twitching of lips, nostrils and ears.
- Muscle tremors, particularly neck and limbs, followed by muscular rigidity.
- Jerky, stiff movement, with progressive incoordination, loss of balance with frequent falling.
- Apparent blindness, head pressing.
- Convulsions, paralysis, recumbency and death.

Postmortem findings

- Non-suppurative encephalomyelitis.

Diagnosis

- Serology – detection of IgM antibody is diagnostic but some animals have little antibody while clinically ill.
- Virus isolation from brain tissue.

Treatment

- None.

Control

- Vaccination with louping ill vaccine (Coopers Pitman-Moore), a single injection repeated every 2 years.

Public health considerations

- The high titres of virus excreted in goats' milk provide a potential zoonotic risk. Goats in tick areas should be vaccinated to reduce the possible risk to the public.

2–7 months

Trauma (qv)

Delayed swayback

See Chapter 5.

Spinal abscess

Coccidiosis

See Chapter 13.

Kids with severe coccidiosis sometimes show nervous signs – dullness, depression, head pressing, opisthotonos and death.

CAE

See Chapter 6.

Caprine arthritis encephalitis virus can produce neurological signs in the kid (*caprine leucoencephalitis*) and the adult goat – neurological signs have *not* been reported in the UK.

Juvenile form: kids 2–4 months old

Consistent with upper motor neurone disease involving an ascending infection of the spinal cord. Spinal reflexes frequently intact (cf Swayback).

Clinical signs

- Pyrexia or fluctuating high temperature (*not* always).
- Bright and alert, good appetite until recumbent.
- Tremor.
- Initial lameness and ataxia, progressing over a number of days to hemiplegia or tetraplegia, circling, hyperaesthesia, blindness and recumbency with torticollis (indicates disease involving higher centres, particularly midbrain).

Treatment

- None.

Adult form

Neurological signs often preceded by other clinical signs of CAE (arthritis, pneumonia, mastitis) and may be complicated by the painful arthritic lesions. In the absence of arthritis, may resemble listeriosis.

Clinical signs

- Knuckling of fetlocks, circling, progressing to paresis and paralysis.

Laboratory tests

- Serology; kids often seronegative at this age although passive maternal antibodies may be detected. Test kid's dam and any goat used to supply kid with milk.
- CSF analysis – generally elevated white cell count (many mononuclear cells) and protein level.

Postmortem findings

- Perivascular mononuclear cell infiltration, and perivascular demyelination in the white matter.
- Gross lesions may be visible in the spinal cord as swollen brownish areas of malacia that are usually unilateral.

7 months–adult

Infectious disease

Listeriosis

Aetiology

- *Listeria monocytogenes*, a gram positive, β-haemolytic bacillus.

Transmission

- By ingestion of the organism which is resistant in the environment surviving in the soil and water for several months and in silage for over 5 years.
- Direct contact with the products of abortion by ingestion or via the conjunctivae.
- Venereal transmission may occur.
- Latent carriers exist and when stressed may excrete the organism.
- The incubation period at 10–15 days is generally shorter than in sheep.

Clinical signs

(1) Encephalitis

- Depression, anorexia, pyrexia.
- Facial paralysis, drooping of ears and eyelids (often asymmetrical), protruding of tongue, drooling of saliva.
- Dysphagia – cud remains in mouth.
- Head tilt, nystagmus, circling, head pressing.
- Progressively incoordinate movement – knuckling, rigidity, paresis.
- Recumbency, opisthotonos, convulsions.
- Death (mortality rate 3–30%).

NB (a) Very acute encephalitis does not always present as the 'circling disease' more typical of sheep. Goats may be presented as dull and incoordinate with death occurring in as little as 6 hours. The disease may be mistaken for hypocalcaemia or even pneumonia.

(b) Abortion and encephalitis occur in the same goat more commonly than is the case for sheep.

(2) Sudden death

- Because the disease in goats may be very acute – goats are much more susceptible to listerial encephalitis than sheep – listeriosis should be considered in the differential diagnosis of sudden death (see Chapter 18).

(3) Septicaemia

- Lethargy, pyrexia (41°C) and bloody diarrhoea in young animals with signs lasting from a few days to several weeks.

(4) Abortion

- See Chapter 2.

(5) Keratoconjunctivitis

- See Chapter 19.

(6) Metritis/vaginal discharge.

Diagnosis

- Physical and neurological examination – clinical signs vary depending on areas of brain involved but include mostly upper motor neurone signs involving ipsilateral limbs.
- Laboratory tests
  (a) examination of CSF – elevated white cells (mononuclear cells and neutrophils)
      elevated protein content
  (b) examination of urine – glucosuria, ketonuria
  (c) examination of paired serum samples
  (d) culture and identification of *L.monocytogenes* from brain, liver, spleen, kidney and heart, fetal stomach, uterine discharges, milk and placenta.
- Postmortem examination
    gross brain lesions may be minimal, possibly congested meninges and oedema
    suppurative meningoencephalitis; microabscesses in the brain stem usually unilateral, vasomeningeal cellular infiltration.

Treatment

- Early treatment with high doses of antibiotics (ampicillin or trimethoprim/sulphonamides), intravenous where possible, and with maintenance doses for at least 7 days.
- Supportive therapy – vitamins, fluids, flunixin meglumine, phenylbutazone or corticosteroids – where indicated.
- It may be advantageous to treat all animals in an affected group with long-acting ampicillin.

Control

- Difficult.
- Avoid soil contaminated feed, particularly silage.
- Ensure good quality silage is made – do not feed mouldy silage, silage with a pH content >5 or an ash content

>70 mg/kg DM; reject silage from damaged bales. Remove any silage not eaten within 24 hours.
- Keep food and water containers clean: avoid faecal contamination.
- Vaccination – experimental studies have yielded variable results. Sheep vaccine available in parts of Europe.

Public health considerations

- Carrier goats may excrete the organism under stress – milk may be infected. Pasteurized cheese has also been implicated in recent outbreaks.

Scrapie

Aetiology

- Scrapie is a progressive fatal degenerative disease of the central nervous system of sheep and goats related to bovine spongiform encephalopathy (BSE), transmissable mink encephalopathy and Creutzfeldt-Jakob disease and Kuru of man. It is caused by a small infectious agent with some of the properties of a virus. Separate strains of the agent exist and the development of clinical disease depends on the scrapie strain as well as on host genetic factors. An age related susceptibility means that maximum opportunity for disease spread is from dam to kid between birth and 9 months of age.

Transmission

Possible routes of transmission are:

- *Doe to kid*
  - (1) *Prenatal?*
    - (a) *transplacental* – unlikely; some evidence that snatching kids at birth stops transmission
    - (b) *infection of egg* – embryo transplant studies suggest egg transmission is unlikely.
  - (2) *Postnatal* – licking or sucking, fetal membranes.
- *Lateral*
  - (1) Oral
    - (a) by *ingestion of fetal membranes* (known to be heavily infected)
    - (b) *contamination* of pasture, troughs, etc. (but very low levels of infection in body fluids)
    - (c) by *goat feed containing scrapie-infected meat and bone meal* as with BSE in cattle.

(2) Conjunctival?
(3) Direct infection via needles, etc.?

Clinical signs

- Because of the long incubation period, the disease is rarely seen in goats less than 2 years old. Animals infected close to parturition often first show clinical signs at around 3 or 4 years of age.
- Two forms of scrapie, *pruritic* and *nervous* have been described in the goat but there is considerable overlap between the two forms and many naturally infected animals show a combination of pruritic and neurological signs.
- Initially, clinical signs may be very non-specific – behavioural changes, increased excitability, lethargy or apprehension, weight loss despite a good appetite, reduced milk yield, and in some animals more specific signs may not become apparent, at least for a considerable period. Most goats, however, progressively show more obvious signs.

  (1) Pruritic signs
  scratching with hind feet
  rubbing poll, withers and back
  nibbling abdomen, sides or udder when touched
  biting at limbs

  (2) Neurological signs
  behavioural changes
  hyperaesthesia
  tremor of the head and neck or whole body
  incoordination, particularly of hind limbs
  postural and gait changes, e.g. highstepping fore limbs
  ataxia
  ears pricked, tail cocked and carried over back
  excessive salivation with strings of saliva at mouth
  cud dropping
  ocular changes – nystagmus; apparent blindness
  death in weeks or months.

Diagnosis

- Clinical signs.
- Histological lesions of the central nervous system.

Postmortem findings

- No obvious gross pathology.

- Histologically there is vacuolation of nerve cells in the medulla, pons and midbrain, with interstitial spongy degeneration.

Louping ill – (qv)

Tetanus – (qv)

CAE – (qv)

Pseudorabies (Aujesky's disease)

Aetiology

- Herpes virus occurring mainly in pigs but occasionally in goats, other ruminants, dogs and cats in contact with pigs.

Clinical signs

- Intense pruritus.
- Mania, ataxia.
- Paralysis, death.

Diagnosis

- Clinical signs.
- History of exposure to pigs.
- Viral isolation; fluorescent antibody test.

Treatment

- None.

Rabies

Aetiology

- Rhabdovirus virus spread by bite of an infected animal.

Clinical signs

- Two forms:
  (1) Furious form – less common. Hyperexcitability, ataxia, sexual excitement, mania, hoarse voice, paralysis, death.
  (2) Dumb form – clinically similar to listeriosis. Ataxia, swaying of hindquarters, tenesmus, paralysis of anus, salivation, loss of voice, paralysis, death.

Postmortem findings

- Histopathology shows Negri bodies in brain tissue.

Metabolic disease

Cerebrocortical necrosis (CCN, polioencephalomalacia)

Aetiology

- Thiamine (vitamin B_1) deficiency. Thiamine (vitamin B_1) is usually produced in adequate amounts by ruminal microflora. Deficiency can arise by:

  (1) Thiaminase type 1 production by ruminal bacteria – possibly following ingestion of mouldy or fungal contaminated feed or acidosis resulting in changes in rumen microflora.
  (2) Prolonged diarrhoea, e.g. coccidiosis.
  (3) Drug therapy, e.g. thiabendazole, levamisole and amprolium
  NB Take care when treating diarrhoea – may exacerbate CCN.
  (4) Plant thiaminase ingestion, e.g. bracken poisoning (*Pteridium aquilinum*).

Clinical signs

- Generally young animals, older animals also affected.
- Stargazing, ataxia, nystagmus, blindness (normal pupillary light reflexes, dorsomedial strabismus) head pressing, collapse ± convulsions and opisthotonus.
- Severe but transient diarrhoea.
- Afebrile (except during convulsions).
- Death 1–2 days after onset of clinical signs.

Laboratory tests

- Estimates of thiamine levels can be made:
  (1) indirectly by erythrocyte transketolase assay on heparinized blood.
  (2) directly on samples of frozen brain, liver or heart.
- Thiaminase levels can be estimated in frozen faecal or rumen samples.
- CSF may show slightly elevated protein levels and white cell count (but relatively acellular compared to pituitary abscess syndrome or listeriosis).
- Urine may test positive for glucose due to hyperglycaemia.

Postmortem findings

- Cerebral oedema produces a swollen brain with disparity in colour between the normal grey of the cerebellar grey matter and the comparatively pale or yellowish grey cerebral cortex.
- Cut surface of cerebral cortex exhibits auto-fluorescence under ultraviolet light.

Treatment

- Thiamine twice daily initially i.v. then i.m. (5–10 mg/kg). The response to thiamine is diagnostic but will only be successful if treatment is commenced early; in more advanced cases, there may be residual brain damage and blindness.
- Unaffected animals in a group should be treated as a preventative.
- Support therapy with corticosteroids, diuretics and hypertonic i.v. drips may aid recovery by reducing the cerebral oedema.

Hypocalcaemia (milk fever)

Aetiology

- There is a fall in the serum calcium and phosphorus levels in all goats at kidding due to the onset of lactation; a greater fall occurs in goats which develop the disease around parturition due to a failure in the calcium homeostatic mechanisms to meet the increased demand for calcium.
- In heavy milking goats, an absolute deficiency of calcium at any stage of lactation will precipitate the disease.

Incidence

- Frank clinical signs are *not* common in the UK, although it is probable that subclinical disease is more widespread and many goats will benefit from calcium therapy when presented with other periparturient diseases such as mastitis, metritis, etc.
- The disease is commonest in young, high yielding first kidders the first few weeks after parturition but may occur in late pregnancy, during parturition and *at any stage of lactation* particularly in heavy milkers and in any age of adult goat. Older goats are more likely to suffer from hypocalcaemia around and during parturition.

Clinical signs

- Often only slight tremors and twitching with some hyperexcitability and slight ataxia, or even lethargy, inappetence and poor milk yield with no obvious nervous signs.
- More severe cases show marked ataxia and incoordination or fits followed by paresis, paraplegia, recumbency and coma which may last several hours.
- An eclamptic form occasionally occurs during lactation, e.g. after a change to better pasture with pyrexia (41.1°C) marked muscular tremors, excitement, rapid panting respirations, collapse and death. *All recumbent or comatose goats should be treated as potentially hypocalcaemic and given calcium.*

Diagnosis

- Clinical signs.
- Rapid response to calcium therapy.
- Serum calcium measurements (normal 2.2–2.6 mmol/litre).

Treatment

- 80–100 ml of calcium borogluconate with 20% (or better calcium borogluconate, magnesium and phosphorus) slowly i.v., s.c. or half by each route. The response to calcium by the s.c. route is very rapid in the goat and may be preferable if the goat is stressed by handling.
- Relapses may occur in which case extra phosphorus as well as calcium may be beneficial.

NB   Many toxic conditions, e.g. enterotoxaemia and mastitis may show a temporary response to calcium therapy.

Hypomagnesaemia (grass tetany)

Aetiology

- Heavy milking goats grazing lush heavily fertilized grass may receive a diet deficient in magnesium. The disease usually occurs fairly early in lactation soon after starting to graze rich pasture. Pregnant goats on poor pasture in early spring may also develop the disease.

Incidence

- The disease is of sporadic occurrence in the UK because most high yielding goats are, at least in part, zero grazed and supplied with hay, browsings and concentrates.

Clinical signs

- *Acute*
  excitement, tremors, twitching of facial muscles
  hyperaesthesia, aimless wandering, falling over, frothing at the mouth
  convulsions, death
  some animals may be found dead.
- *Subclinical*
  inappetence, apprehension, milk yield decreased, mild ataxia, may convulse in response to noise or handling
  may be spontaneous recovery or progression to acute phase
- *Chronic*
  other animals in an affected herd may show poor growth, reduced milk yield and dullness due to low serum magnesium levels.

Diagnosis

- Clinical signs.
- Response to treatment.
- Serum magnesium levels (normal 0.83–1.6 mmol/l).

Treatment

- 80–100 ml calcium borogluconate 20% with magnesium and phosphorus i.v. or s.c., plus 100 ml of magnesium sulphate 25% s.c.
- Oral maintenance dose of at least 7 g of calcinated magnesite or equivalent while dietary imbalances are corrected.

Prevention

- Correct diet – good quality fibre, adequate energy plus adequate magnesium (supplement where necessary, e.g. Rumbol magnesium sheep bullets (Agrimin)).
- Avoid grazing heavily fertilized pastures.

Transit tetany

Aetiology

- Combined hypocalcaemia/hypomagnesaemia brought on by stress, particularly transport but also by late pregnancy, fear, etc.
- May occur in castrated males.

Clinical signs

- As for acute hypomagnesaemia.

Treatment

- As for acute hypomagnesaemia.

Periparturient toxaemia

See Chapter 8.

Does with *pregnancy toxaemia* and *acetonaemia* occasionally show nervous signs – ataxia, tremors around the head and ears, reduced vision or blindness, head pressing, stargazing and eventually recumbency, coma and death.

Does with *postparturient toxaemia* (fatty liver syndrome) generally only show nervous signs terminally when starvation results in recumbency and coma.

Space-occupying lesions of the brain

Cerebral abscess

- Bacterial infection often with *C.pyogenes, Staphylococcus aureus* or *Fusobacterium necrophorum;* often follows fight wounds in male goats.

Clinical signs

- Variable; may be associated with meningitis or act as a space-occupying lesion with head tilt, visual defects, circling (with head turned towards side of lesion) etc. Brain stem compression may cause ataxia, weakness or asymmetric pupil size.
- CSF changes variable – often increased white cell count (neutrophils).

Coenuriasis (gid)

Aetiology

- Intracranial pressure from cyst of the tapeworm *Taenia multiceps, Coenurus cerebralis.*

Clinical signs

- Clinical signs depend on the location of the cyst and the pressure it exerts on the surrounding brain tissue. Pressure on the cerebral hemispheres results in incoordination, blindness, head tilt, head pressing, circling, stargazing. Gait abnormalities occur when the cerebellum is involved. Skull softening as a result of bone rarefaction may occur when the cyst is superficial.

Diagnosis

- Intradermal gid test – 0.1 ml cyst fluid injected into caudal fold beneath tail or shaved area of skin on neck; 0.1 ml sterile water used as control. Skin thickening at test site within 24 hours classified as positive. Not very reliable.
- Serology and haematology of no diagnostic use; CSF – increased white cell count particularly eosinophils and mononuclear cells.
- Surgery or postmortem examination

Treatment

- Surgical removal of the cyst, when it can be located by skull softening, under sedation and local anaesthesia or general anaesthetic. Skin incised and bone removed with trephine or scalpel blade. After the dura mater is penetrated, the cyst will often bulge through and can be removed by applying negative suction pressure by syringe or pipette.
- Where there is no skull softening but the cyst site can be approximately located by detailed neurological examination, ultrasound examination via a trephine site may aid localization.
- Radiography can also be used but interpretation of the results is difficult.

Control

- Regular treatment of all dogs on the farm for tapeworm.

Pituitary abscess syndrome

Aetiology

- Abscessation of the pituitary gland following lymphatic or blood-borne infection often with *C.pyogenes* but also many other gram positive (*Streptococcus, Staphylococcus, Actinomyces*) and gram negative (*Fusobacterium, Bacteroides, Pasteurella, Pseudomonas, Actinobacillus*) bacteria from another infected focus in the body, e.g. mastitis, arthritis, lung abscess, sinusitis or intracranial damage with secondary sepsis after fighting.

Pressure by the enlarging abscess acts as a space-occupying lesion affecting the adjacent areas of the brain and brain stem and producing various neurological signs depending on the extent of the abscess. Cranial nerve functions are progressively affected, usually asymmetrically.

Incidence

- Generally adult animals; more commonly males.

Clinical signs

Varying clinical signs but commonly:

- Anorexia, depression.
- Bradycardia (see below).
- Dysphagia.
- Head pressing.
- Blindness (pupillary light reflexes often absent; ventrolateral strabismus, cf. cerebrocortical necrosis).
- Nystagmus.
- Ataxia, opisthotonus, recumbency.
- Death.

NB (1) The progressive nature of the neurological signs means that repeat neurological examinations and assessment of cranial nerve function is important for diagnosis. (2) *Bradycardia* is an uncommon finding in the goat but occurs in the *pituitary abscess syndrome* and other *space-occupying lesions* of the brain because pressure on the hypothalamus causes increased vagal tone. Bradycardia may also occur in *severe milk fever, hypothermia, hypoglycaemia, botulism* and *trauma* to the head.

Laboratory findings

- CSF – elevated white cell count (mostly neutrophils) elevated protein level.
- Haematology – not diagnostic; fibrinogen and globulin often elevated.

Postmortem findings

- Pituitary abscess – generally evident grossly, occasionally only on histopathological examination.
- Generally a chronic infection elsewhere in the body.

- Histopathology shows coagulative and liquefactive necrosis of the pituitary gland, particularly the adenohypophysis with neutrophil and some mononuclear cell infiltration.
- Culture of abscess sample yields pure or mixed culture of aerobic bacteria.

Treatment

- None.

Oestrus ovis

Oestrus ovis, the sheep and goat nasal fly, deposits larvae around the nostrils. The larvae normally migrate to the nasal passages and then the frontal sinuses. Clinical signs are usually limited to panic when the flies are laying and a mucopurulent discharge when the larvae are in the nasal passages and sinuses. Larvae may rarely migrate via the ethmoid bones to brain producing clinical signs as for *Coenurus cerebralis*. Larvae may also occasionally enter the eye or nasolacrimal system causing conjunctivitis.

Space-occupying lesions of the spinal cord

Although more common in kids (qv) *spinal meningitis, abscessation* and *vertebral osteomyelitis* may occur in adult animals producing varying degrees of paraparesis or tetraparesis.

CSF – variable, often increased white cell count (neutrophils).

Treatment should be based where possible on culture and sensitivity of the CSF or use long-term broad spectrum antibiotic therapy.

Tumours, e.g. lymphosarcoma, meningioma and *Coenurus cerebralis cysts* (qv) may rarely act as space-occupying lesions of the spinal cord.

Cerebrospinal nematodiasis – aberrant spinal cord migration of any nematode may occasionally cause neurological signs, generally referrable to spinal cord disease.

CSF shows elevated white cells (mainly eosinophils and mononuclear cells) and protein levels.

Treatment with ivermectin (Ivomec injection, MSD) and dexamethasone may be successful if combined with adequate supportive care.

Trauma (qv)

Trauma to the head and neck should always be considered, particularly in male goats running together or tethered animals.

Vestibular disease

Otitis media/interna

Occur as sequelae to otitis externa or following rhinitis and pharyngitis; or via haematogenous spread.

Clinical signs

- Head tilt, circling towards side of affected ear, nystagmus with fast component directed away from the affected ear.
- Eye drop on the affected side.
- Facial paralysis.

Ear mite infection (psoroptic mange)

See Chapter 10.

Hepatic encephalopathy

Uncommon; severe hepatic insufficiency may result in lethargy, depression and neurological signs such as behavioural changes, ataxia, tremors, fits, convulsions and coma.

Halothane induced acute hepatic necrosis has been described as producing depression, lethargy, salivation, head pressing, chewing motions, icterus and recumbency.

Poisonings

A variety of drugs, plants and chemicals can be neurotoxic.

Lead poisoning

Aetiology

- Lead from old painted wood (check partitions, doors, etc.), car batteries, motor oil, etc.

Clinical signs

- Blindness (normal pupillary light reflexes), head pressing, ataxia.

- Abdominal pain, anorexia, weight loss.
- Diarrhoea, tenesmus.

Laboratory tests

- Blood lead estimation.
- Basophilic stippling of erythrocytes stained with Wright's stain.
- Kidney or liver lead levels – >4 ppm.
- CSF – acellular.

Postmortem findings

- Cerebral oedema.
- Mucoid enterocolitis.

Treatment

- Calcium disodium versenate 20% 75 mg/kg, i.v. or s.c. in divided doses every few hours for 3 or 4 days.

NB Poisoning with other heavy metals such as *arsenic* and *mercury* may occasionally occur giving neurological signs such as incoordination, blindness, muscle tremors and convulsions, together with abdominal pain and diarrhoea.

Plant poisoning

See Chapter 20.

Unlikely to produce nervous signs in goats in the UK. Rape (*Brassica rapus*) can produce blindness, head pressing and violent excitement. Bracken (*Pteridium aquilinum*), although unlikely to induce a thiamine deficiency under normal conditions where ruminal synthesis of thiamine is adequate, might exacerbate or precipitate cerebrocortical necrosis (qv). Oxalate poisoning which can produce ataxia, muscle tremor paralysis and death might by produced by eating large amounts of rhubarb or common sorrel. Fool's parsley (*Aethusa cynapuim*) can cause indigestion, panting and ataxia. Cherry laurel (*Prunus laurocerasus*) causes cyanide poisoning with animals often being found dead. Less severe cases show dyspnoea, staggering gait, jerky movements and convulsions. Laburnum (*L.anagyroides*) and hemlock (*Corium maculatum*) contain nicotine-like alkaloids resulting in rapid respirations, salivation, excitement and muscle tremors followed by depression, incoordination, convulsions and death. Ragwort produces an hepatic neurotoxicity.

Organophosphate poisoning

Exposure to organophosphates, e.g. dips or drenches.

Clinical signs

- Abdominal pain, inappetence, incoordination, diarrhoea, muscular tremors, dyspnoea, paralysis, convulsions, coma and death.

Treatment

- Atropine 1 mg/kg slowly i.v.

Rafoxanide

Rafoxanide (Flukanide Drench, MSD) has a much lower safety margin in goats (4–6 times) than sheep (20 times). Overdosage may cause degeneration and oedema of the retina, optic tract and related areas of the CNS and death.

Urea (hyperammonaemia)

- Overfeeding of urea in rations.
- Abdominal pain, muscle tremor, ataxia, hyperaesthesia.
- Mydriasis, convulsions and death.

Treatment

- Vinegar orally as an acidifying agent.

Epilepsy

A single case of partial epilepsy has been reported in a Nubian goat.

Further reading

General

Barlow, R. M. (1987) Differential diagnosis of nervous diseases of goats. *Goat Vet. Soc. J.*, **8** (2), 73–76

Baxendell, S. A. (1984) Caprine nervous diseases. *Proc. Univ. Sydney, Post Grad. Comm. Vet. Sci.*, **73**, 333–342

Brewer, B. D. (1983) Neurologic disease of sheep and goats. *Vet. Clin. North Amer.: Large Animal Practice*, **5** (3), November 1983, 677–700

Thompson, K. G. (1985) Nervous diseases of goats. *Proc. Course in Goat Husbandry and Medicine, Massey University*, November 1985, 152–161

Listeriosis

Harwood, D. G. (1988) Listeriosis in goats. *Goat Vet. Soc. J.*, **10** (1), 1–4

Meningitis

Jamison, J. M. and Prescott, J. F. (1987) Bacterial meningitis in large animals Part I. *Comp. Cont. Ed. Pract. Vet.*, **9** (12), F399–F406

Jamison, J. M. and Prescott, J. F. (1988) Bacterial meningitis in large animals Part II. *Comp. Cont. Ed. Pract. Vet.*, **10** (2), 225–231

Disbudding meningoencephalitis

Wright, H. J., Adams, D. S. and Trigo, F. J. (1983) Meningoencephalitis after hot iron disbudding of goat kids. *VMSAC*, **78** (4), 599–601

Scrapie

Kimberlin, R. H. (1981) Scrapie. *Brit. Vet. J.*, **134** (1), 105–112

Cerebrocortical necrosis

Baxendell, S. A. (1984) Cerebrocortical necrosis. *Proc. Univ. Sydney Post Grad. Comm. Vet. Sci.*, **73**, 503–507

Smith, M. C. (1979) Polioencephalomalacia in goats. *JAVMA*, **174** (12), 1328–1332

Caprine arthritis encephalitis

Adams, D. S., Klevjer-Anderson, P., Carlson, J. L., McGuire, T. C. and Gorham, J. R. (1983) Transmission and control of CAE virus. *Am. J. Vet. Res.*, **44** (9), 1670–1675

Dawson, M. (1987) Caprine arthritis encephalitis. *In Practice*, Jan. 1987, 8–11

Knight, A. P. and Jokinen, M. P. (1982) Caprine arthritis encephalitis. *Comp. Cont. Ed. Pract. Vet.*, **4** (6), S263–S269

Metabolic and nutritional diseases

Andrews, A. H. (1985) Some metabolic conditions in the doe. *Goat Vet. Soc. J.*, **6** (2), 70–72

Merrall, M. (1985) Nutritional and metabolic diseases. *Proc. Course in Goat Husbandry and Medicine, Massey University*, November 1985, 126–131

Pinsent, J. and Cottom, D. S. (1987) Metabolic diseases of goats. *Goat Vet. Soc. J.*, **8** (1), 40–42

Enzootic ataxia

Inglis, D. M., Gilmour, J. S. and Murray, I. S. (1986) A farm investigation into swayback in a herd of goats and the result of administration of copper needles. *Vet. Rec.*, **118**, 657–660

Whitelaw, A. (1985) Copper deficiency in cattle and sheep. *In Practice*, May 1985, 98–100

Coenuriasis

Harwood, D. G. (1986) Metacestode disease in goats. *Goat Vet. Soc. J.*, **7** (2), 35–38

Ear mites

Littlejohn, A. I. (1968) Psoroptic mange in the goat. *Vet. Rec.*, **82**, 148–155
Williams, J. F. and Williams, S. F. (1978) Psoroptic ear mites in dairy goats. *JAVMA*, **173** (12), 1582–1583

Tickborne diseases

Reid, H. W. (1986) Tick and tickborne diseases. *Goat Vet. Soc. J.*, **7** (2), 21–25

β-Mannosidosis

Kumar, K., Jones, M. Z., Cunninham, J. G., Kelly, J. A. and Lovell, K. L. (1986) Caprine β-mannosidosis: phenotypic features. *Vet. Rec.*, **118**, 325–327

Pituitary abscess syndrome

Perdrizet, J. and Dinsmore, P. (1986) *Comp. Cont. Ed. Pract. Vet.*, **8** (6), S311–S318

12 Diseases of the mammary gland

Mastitis
'Hard udder'
Udder oedema
Trauma to the udder
Abscesses
Fibrous scar tissue
Pustular dermatitis of the udder
Fly bites
Tumours
Orf
Maiden milkers
'Witch's milk'
Milking males (gynaecomastia)
Milk problems
Teat abnormalities

- Mastitis.
- 'Hard' udder.
- Udder oedema.
- Trauma.
- Abscess.
- Fibrous scar tissue.
- Pustular dermatitis of the udder.
- Fly bites.
- Tumour.
- Orf.
- Maiden milkers.
- 'Witch's milk.
- Milking males.

Milk problems

- Blood in milk ('pink milk').
- Milk leakage.
- Self sucking.
- Milk taint.

Teat abnormalities

- 'Pea' in the teat.
- Supernumerary and abnormal teats.

Mastitis

Inflammation of the mammary gland regardless of cause characterized by physiological, chemical and generally bacteriological changes in milk and by pathological changes in glandular tissue.

Investigation of mastitis

(1) General clinical examination
   - assess severity of systemic infection, degree of pyrexia etc.
(2) Specific udder examination
   - visually and by palpation.
   - compare the two halves.

- heat.
- swelling.
- lumps.
- extent of fibrosis.
- injuries to teats or body of udder.
- superficial inguinal lymph nodes.

(3) Examine milk sample
- use strip cup.
- compare the two halves.
- pus.
- blood.
- clots.
- colour .

In subclinical mastitis the milk may appear grossly normal.

(4) Laboratory tests
- Somatic cell counts
- Whiteside test
- California mastitis test

not reliable in goats because of presence of normal cytoplasmic particles. Infections with known pathogens give comparable results to those in cows but similar results can be obtained from milk samples in which no bacteria can be isolated.

Somatic cell counts useful as *herd* test to monitor subclinical mastitis.

- *Bacteriology on a sterile milk sample*
  Collection of sample: clean teats thoroughly with 70% ethanol, discard foremilk, collect 20 ml of milk from each half in sterile containers; if not tested immediately store at 4°C (can freeze for several weeks if necessary).

Only need to use standard bacterial media (*Mycoplasma* spp. not implicated in mastitis in UK).

Identify bacteria present and carry out antibiotic sensitivity tests.

NB In some types of mastitis, excretion of bacteria is only intermittent, e.g. *Pseudomonas* spp. and chronic *Staph. aureus* mastitis.

Coagulase positive *Staph. aureus* is the commonest cause of caprine mastitis, causing gangrenous, non-gangrenous or subclinical mastitis.

Coagulase negative staphylococci are the most frequently isolated organisms – significance uncertain; probably commensal organisms rather than primary pathogens.

Environmental mastitis caused by organisms, such as *E.coli*, *Pseudomonas* spp. and *Klebsiella* spp. is rare; most frequently seen as subclinical mastitis.

Many bacteria such as *Streptococcus* spp. and *Pasteurella haemolytica* occasionaly cause mastitis. *Yersinia pseudotuberculosis* has been isolated from milk of an aborting goat. Fungi and yeasts such as *Candida albicans* are occasionally isolated.

Mycoplasma spp. have not been reported as causing mastitis in the UK but they are an important problem in many other countries including a number of EEC members. *Mycoplasma agalactiae* causes contagious agalactia; *Mycoplasma mycoides subspecies mycoides* is implicated in contagious pleuropneumonia and a variety of serious syndromes. *Mycoplasma putrefaciens* causes agalactia.

Corynebacterium pyogenes and *C. pseudotuberculosis* cause mastitis in herds outwith the UK where the organisms are present.

Clinical mastitis

Peracute or gangrenous mastitis

Aetiology

- Commonly *Staph.aureus* infection following a slight injury to the teat at any stage of lactation: occasionally *E.coli*.

Clinical signs

- Marked pyrexia in early stages, often progressing to a toxaemia with subnormal temperature and death; may present as sudden death.
- Udder hard, hot swollen and painful; minimal thin, bloody serous fluid from teat.
- Pain syndrome – teeth grinding, rapid pulse.

Prognosis

- Guarded; if the animal survives, the affected half becomes gangrenous, cold and clammy, turning blue through purple to black and eventually sloughing.

Treatment

- Economically treatment is often not worthwhile.
  In a pet goat or where the goat is to be kept for breeding.
- Intensive intravenous antibiotic therapy (ampicillin, tetracyclines etc.), flunixin meglumine (Finadyne, Schering Plough) and supportive therapy with intravenous fluids, rugs and human company are essential.
- As the udder sloughs and the teat is lost milk may still be produced by the dorsal portion and mastectomy may be necessary.
- Alternatively, infusion of Lugol's iodine or acriflavine under local anaesthesia can be used to dry up the affected side.
- Mastectomy can also be considered in male goats.

Acute mastitis

Aetiology

- A number of different bacteria.

Clinical signs

- Pyrexia, anorexia, lethargy.
- Udder hard swollen and painful.
- Milk yield decreased; milk consistency changed.
- Often thin and watery with clots.

Prognosis

- Clinical recovery may result in subclinical disease or fibrosis and atrophy of the half.

Treatment

- Broad spectrum antibiotics, parenteral and intramammary until results of laboratory tests are known.

Mild clinical mastitis

Aetiology

- A number of different bacteria.

Clinical signs

- Only very mild or no systemic signs.
- Local udder reaction, possibly with slightly swollen half,

small clots or pus in milk; milk often thinner than usual. Most milk samples presented for testing are from goats that are not clinically ill but where there are a few clots or crystals in the milk, poor keeping quality of milk, milk taint or curdling on boiling milk.

Terminal fibrosis and atrophy

The endpoint of most forms of mastitis is fibrosis and atrophy of the affected mammary tissue as healing takes place. Lesions may be confined to localized areas or may involve the greater part of the half. Fibrosis produces palpable induration and decreased milk yield. Contraction of the fibrous tissue produces visible and palpable atrophy.

Pockets of infection may remain and form abscesses.

Subclinical mastitis

Udder and milk secretion are clinically normal although fibrosis and atrophy may be present from a previous clinical infection. There is usually some reduction in milk yield which may be economically significant. There may also be a reduction in the levels of butter fat and no fat solids and a decreased keepability.

The true level of subclinical mastitis is unknown although surveys have suggested that between 4 and 6% of halves are affected with known pathogens.

Intramammary antibiotic treatment

At the present time, there are no intramammary preparations which are specifically licensed for goats, available in the UK. Experimental work shows clearly that clearance times of antibiotic preparations from the mammary gland of goats may differ markedly from those from bovine mammary glands. In some cases, e.g. oxytetracycline, erythromycin, rapid elimination of drug may occur to the extent that therapeutic efficiency may be compromised. With other preparations, e.g. amoxycillin trihydrate/potassium clavulanate/prednisolone (Synulox LC, Beecham Animal Health), a withholding time approximately double that for cows, is required. With all preparations used outwith data sheet recommendations *a minimum 7 day withdrawal period* should be imposed for milk.

In addition, the nozzles of some intramammary preparations are too large to be inserted easily into goat teats with the resultant risk of introducing infection or traumatizing the teat. Long-acting preparations, e.g. cephacetrite sodium (Vetimast, Ciba-Geigy) or cefoperazone (Pathocef, Pfizer), may thus be useful in that only a single tube need be inserted and prolonged action can be obtained within a 7 day withholding period.

Dry-goat therapy

- Use whenever there has been clinical mastitis or evidence of subclinical mastitis during the lactation; many infections, e.g. *Staph. aureus* are easier to treat during the dry period.
- ? Use routinely; danger of introducing infection when inserting tubes (especially with inexperienced owner or goat with small teat orifice).
- Always thoroughly clean teat with spirit before insertion and use a teat dip after insertion.
- Always use a seperate tube for each half.

Drying off

- An 8-week dry period before parturition as with cows is recommended. Many high yielding goats will still be giving substantial quantities of milk (4.5 + litres daily) at this stage.
- Stop milking abruptly – in high yielders, udder may become quite large until the pressure stops milk production, but within a few days the udder will shrink and become softer. Pressure of milk causes an inflammatory response so leucocytes collect in the udder helping to prevent infection. Reducing concentrates for a few days before drying off may help reduce milk production in very high yielders. Milking only once daily for a week before drying off will help.
- *Never* partially milk out an udder as this increases the susceptibility to infection.
- Teat dipping for a week after stopping milking will help prevent infection during drying off.

'Hard udder'

- A firm, swollen udder in freshly kidded goats (often first kidders).
- Little milk, production with poor milk let down.
- Non-responsive to treatments for oedematous udders, e.g. diuretics.

- Milk appears normal with no evidence of bacterial mastitis.
- Increased milk production and softening of the udder occurs after about a week but milk production remains suboptimum throughout the lactation because of the indurative changes in the udder tissue.

In the UK at least, the condition appears to be part of the CAE complex. All goats seen by the author with this condition have been CAE seropositive and since the widespread introduction of CAE control measures the incidence has fallen to zero.

Udder oedema

Occasionally, the normal physiological oedema of the udder which occurs prior to parturition is excessive resulting in an udder which is hard and swollen. Unlike the 'hard udder' syndrome, milk production is not severely affected. In the UK, although some goats may need milking before kidding to ease the udder, it is extremely rare to have to resort to any further treatment. In contrast the condition is reported to be common in British Alpines, particularly first kidders, in Australia suggesting that some factor other than a normal physiological process is involved. In severe cases of oedema, hot compresses, liniments and frequent stripping may be necessary together with 5 ml of Lasix (Hoechst) or other diuretic twice daily for 3 days.

Trauma to the udder

Traumatic injury to the teats and udder associated with butting and being trodden on are common and may result in large painful swellings, possibly accompanied by mastitis. Any wounds should be carefully treated and antibiotic cover given to prevent the occurrence of mastitis.

Gangrenous mastitis commonly results from quite small abrasions near the teat tip.

Abscesses

Abscesses in the udder may arise from mastitic episodes or from penetrating lesions to the udder. Deep abscesses are not possible to treat, abscesses just below the skin of the udder can be satisfactorily drained.

Fibrous scar tissue

Fibrous lumps arise as a sequel to mastitis or trauma. Because they are an obvious fault in the show ring, owners resort to numerous methods to try to get rid of them. Topical applications of anti-inflammatory creams, herbal remedies etc. will reduce the size of surface lumps but the most successful treatment is cold laser treatment, initially twice weekly, then weekly.

Pustular dermatitis of the udder

See Staphylococcal dermatitis (Chapter 10).

Fly bites

Biting flies may produce quite severe lesions superficially resemblng staphylococcal dermatitis on the udder. Topical creams and washes will ease the lesions.

Tumours

See Chapter 9.

Orf

See Chapter 9.

Maiden milkers

Many kids and goatlings from heavy milking strains show udder development and milk production particularly during the summer months. The vast majority of these animals do *not* require milking – milking stimulates production of more milk necessitating more regular milking, possibly predisposing to mastitis and acting as a nutritional drain on a growing animal. In well grown, well fed animals feed reduction may help control milk production. Milking is only necessary if the amount of milk makes the goat uncomfortable – the udder should be completely emptied as partial milking predisposes to infection; teats should be dipped after milking.

'Witch's milk'

Newborn kids occasionally show mammary development and milk production. No treatment is necessary.

Milking males (gynaecomastia)

Many males from high yielding families, particularly British Saanen and Saanen males, show mammary development and some degree of milk production during the summer months. For this reason, and to limit the risk of laminitis, the protein and energy level of feed should be reduced during the summer. In most males, dietary management will control mammary development without resorting to milking. However, regular checks should be made as gangrenous mastitis is not an uncommon sequel in these animals. The fertility of males with mammary development is not affected.

Milk problems

Blood in the milk ('pink milk')

Haemorrhage into the udder from a damaged blood vessel occurs most commonly in first kidders in the first few days after kidding as the udder adapts to milk production and the stresses of regular milking. It may also occur at other times during lactation, particularly if the goat is milked by someone other than the regular attendant. The degree of haemorrhage determines whether the milk is coloured pink or there is merely a pink sediment after the milk has been allowed to stand.

Culture of a sterile milk sample will confirm the absence of infection in these cases – bloody milk is not a common sign of mastitis.

Treatment is usually not necessary, the condition being self-limiting in a few days.

Milk leakage

Milk will sometimes leak from a teat, particularly at the junction between the teat and the udder, probably due to a thinning of the skin in response to pressure from milking. The condition is usually self-limiting – care should be taken to avoid the affected area when milking. More severe leaks may require suturing.

Self sucking

A quite common problem, which once started is very difficult to stop. A variety of preventative devices can be tried – udder bags, Elizabethan collars, noxious sprays such as Bitter Apple, teat tape (3m) etc. – but many chronic suckers are culled.

Milk taint

Investigation of milk taint

Initial assessment

- Individual or group of animals involved
  – generally an individual animal problem.
- Recent or persistent problem.
- Machine/hand milking – technique; relief milkers.
- Dairy hygiene and practice.
- Storage of milk.
- Type of taint
  'goaty' or not
  obvious before tasting or only after tasting
  present as soon as milked or develops over a few hours.

(1) *Herd problem*
   Consider:

- *Feed taint* – kale, turnips, swedes, garlic, cow parsley, camomile etc. (See Chapter 20).
  Action – identify possible sources of taint, house animals and zero graze on hay rather than green plants.
- *Genetic factors* – certain goats have a high natural lipase enzyme activity causing release of fatty acids, particularly caproic acid.
  Action – identify particular families of goats involved.
- B_{12} *deficiency*
  (a) cobalt deficiency (see Chapter 8)
  (b) helminthiasis (see Chapter 13)
  Results in accumulation of branch chain and odd chain fatty acids and sweet sickly smell.
  Action: worm animals and correct deficiency.
- *Mastitis* – widespread subclinical mastitis may present as a herd problem.
  Action – check milking technique, milking machine maintenance.
- *Poor milking technique* – bacterial contamination of milk.

- *Poor dairy hygiene* – bacterial contamination of milk, inadequate filtration cooling, refrigeration and freezing of milk.
- *Agitation of milk* – releases free fatty acids, particularly caproic acid.
  Action – check pumps and length of milk lines etc.
- *Oxidation*
      (1) exposure to copper or iron (oily/cardboard flavour)
      (2) exposure to sunlight or fluorescent light (flat/burnt flavour).
- *Storage taint* – milk readily picks up strong flavours from other foods etc.

(2) *Individual goat problem*
  - Identify goat.
  - One or both halves of udder involved? – unilateral generally means mastitis, bilateral may be mastitis.
  - Examine udder for lumps, fibrosis, abscess etc.
  - If no bacteria isolated consider other causes of taint as discussed under 'herd problem'.

See Figure 12.1.

Teat abnormalities

'Pea' in the teat

Occasionally a teat obstruction occurs preventing the flow of milk during milking. This is generally a crystal which is too big to pass through the teat orifice but teat lumen granulomas also occur.

Crystals can usually be removed by manipulation and pressure; removal of a granuloma may require teat surgery.

Supernumerary and abnormal teats

Supernumerary and abnormal teats are inherited defects which result in disqualification in show animals. There is thus an ethical consideration before surgical interference is undertaken.

All kids, male and female, should be checked for teat abnormalities at disbudding, but many abnormalities will not become apparent until later.

Discrete, definite supernumerary teats can be removed at disbudding or later. Double teats and fishtail teats are best left intact.

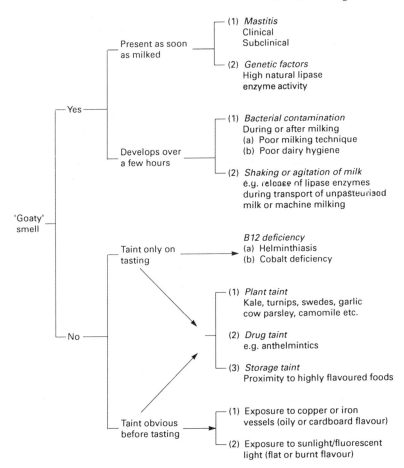

Figure 12.1 Identification of the cause of milk taint (after Mews, A., 1987, *Goat Vet. Soc. J.*, **8** (1), 29–31)

Further reading

Mastitis

Anderson, J. C. (1983) Mastitis in Goats. *Goat Vet. Soc. J.*, 17–20

Baxendell, S. A. (1984) Mastitis. *Proc. Univ. Sydney, Post Grad. Comm. Vet. Sci.*, **73**, 473–483

Cripps, P. (1986) The prevention and control of mastitis in goats. *Goat Vet. Soc. J.*, **7** (2), 48–51

East, N. E. and Birnie, E. F. (1983) Diseases of the udder. *Vet. Clin. North Amer.: Large Animal Practice*, **5** (3), November 1983, 591–600

Manser, P. A. (1985) Mastitis in goats. *Goat Vet. Soc. J.*, **6** (1), 4–6

O'Brien, J. K. (1982) Some aspects of mastitis control in goats. *Goat Vet. Soc. J.*, **3** (1), 13–17

Thornton, D. A. K. (1983) Disease of the mammary gland in goats. *Goat Vet. Soc. J.*, **4** (1), 12–16

Udder conditions

Baxendell, S. A. (1984) Other udder conditions of goats. *Proc. Univ. Sydney Post. Grad. Comm. Vet. Sci.*, **73**, 484–489

Mastectomy

Kerr, H. J. and Wallace, C. E. (1978) Mastectomy in a goat. *VMSAC*, **73** (9), 1177–1181

Milk taint

Baxendell, S. A. (1984) Goat milk taints. *Proc. Univ. Sydney Post. Grad. Comm. Vet. Sci.*, **73**, 493–494

Cousins, C. M. (1981) Milk hygiene and milk taints. *Goat Vet. Soc. J.*, **2** (1), 20–24

Mews, A. (1987) Goat milk taints. *Goat Vet. Soc. J.*, **8** (1), 29–31

Milk hygiene

Ministy of Agriculture, Fisheries and Food, Code of Practice. *The Hygienic Production of Goats' Milk.* MAFF Publications, Alnwick

Department of Agriculture and Fisheries for Scotland, Code of Practice. *The Hygienic Control of Goats' Milk.* Department of Agriculture and Fisheries for Scotland, Edinburgh

13 Diarrhoea

Diarrhoea may be produced by a number of pathogens, toxic substances and nutritional causes.

Birth–4 weeks

Nutritional
Enterotoxigenic *E.coli*
Salmonella spp.
Clostridium perfringens type C
Clostridium perfringens type B
Campylobacter jejuni
Rotavirus
Coronavirus
Cryptosporidium
Strongyloides papillosus

4 weeks–12 weeks

Parasitic gastroenteritis
Coccidiosis
Clostridium perfringens type D
Salmonella
Giardiasis
Nutritional factors
Campylobacter jejuni
Toxic agents

Over 12 weeks

Parasitic gastroenteritis
Coccidiosis
Cl. perfringens type D
Salmonella
Nutritional factors
Toxic agents
Liver disease
Copper deficiency
(Johne's disease)

Initial assessment

The preliminary history should consider:

- Individual or group problem.
- Age of animal(s).
- Weaned or unweaned.
- Acute or chronic problem.
- Nutrition.
  basic diet
  change in diet
  level of concentrate feed (change in batch, excessive amount)
  possible mineral deficiencies.
- In unweaned kids consider:
  on dam or artificially reared
  whole milk or milk replacer
  adlib or restricted feed
  bottle, bowl or machine fed
  type of milk powder, concentration fed and temperature
  one person or number of people responsible for feeding.
- Housing
  individual or group
  deep litter or slats
  mixing of age groups.
- Grazing
  zero grazed
  access to pasture
  pasture rotation.
- Access to toxic materials or plants.
- Preventative medications
  clostridial vaccination
  anthelmintics (frequency, dose rate, accurate assessment of weight?, class of anthelmintic).

Clinical examination

- A full detailed clinical examination is essential to reach an accurate diagnosis.
- Diarrhoeic animals may be hypoproteinaemic with signs of oedema, e.g. bottle jaw, and/or anaemia (see Chapter 17).
- Examine mucous membranes.

- The diarrhoea may be a secondary problem, e.g. in severe toxaemias such as acute mastitis.
- Animals may be bright afebrile and eager to feed or dull, lethargic pyrexic and anorexic.
- Note type and consistency of faeces – colour, mucus, blood.
- Presence or absence of abdominal pain (see also Chapters 14 and 15).
- Signs of dehydration.

Laboratory investigation

- Fresh material is essential for diagnosis. Submission of a live, acutely ill animal may make definitive diagnosis easier.
- A faeces sample (20 to 30 ml) should be collected early in the course of the disease. A faecal swab does not permit diagnosis of anything other than a bacterial infection.
- A complete range of samples for investigation from a live animal includes
    fresh faeces; air dried smears of fresh faeces
    blood samples – EDTA, serum and air dried blood films
    plus at postmortem, freshly fixed sections from all levels of the small and large intestine and unopened loops of intestine.
- The antibody status of kids can be assessed by the use of the zinc sulphate turbidity test on serum.

Treatment

Specific treatments should be instigated where the cause of the diarrhoea is known. In other cases or before a laboratory diagnosis is reached symptomatic treatments may be of value.

(1) Restrict food, particularly concentrates, for 24 hours, gradually increasing to the normal ration as the diarrhoea is controlled and correcting any obvious dietary excess.

   Unweaned kids should be taken off milk for 24 hours and fed water or electrolyte replacer. Reduced quantities of normal strength milk should be offered subsequently.

   NB Feeding milk replacers at less than the recommended concentration is likely to exacerbate the diarrhoea as the milk will not clot properly.

(2) *Fluid therapy* to replace fluid loss and correct the electrolyte balance.

- Oral rehydration therapy with electrolyte solutions (Lectade, Smith Kline Beecham; Life Aid, Norbrook Laboratories).
- Subcutaneous or intravenous balanced electrolyte solutions. 20–120 ml/kg bodyweight given to replace fluid loss depending on the degree of dehydration. Intravenous fluids should be given over a period of 4 or 5 hours.
- The amount of replacement fluid required can be estimated from the percentage fluid loss based on body weight.

% Fluid loss based on body weight	Clinical signs
0–5	Mild, barely detectable
5–10	Moderate, mouth dry, skin remains erect when pinched
10	Severe, body cold, eyes shrunken, comatose

A dehydrated kid requires a weight of fluid equal to the estimated loss due to dehydration, plus a weight of fluid equal to 10% of body weight for daily maintenance. For practical purposes 1 kg = 1 litre of fluid.

Thus a 5 kg kid with 5% fluid loss requires

5% of 5 kg to replace lost fluid = 0.25 kg
plus 10% of 5 kg for maintenance = 0.50 kg
Total fluid required is 0.75 kg = 0.75 l = 750 ml

- Additional bicarbonate is required to combat acidosis in cases of severe diarrhoea, i.e. 150–650 mg of sodium bicarbonate depending on the degree of dehydration (1 teaspoonful = 5 g).

(3) Use non-specific treatments such as kaolin, chalk, bismuth etc.
(4) Use oral antibiotics such as potentiated sulphonamides, neomycin, furazolidone, streptomycin, tetracyclines and framycetin to control oppportunist bacterial pathogens and use parenteral antibiotics if the animal is septicaemic.
(5) Use spasmolytics such as Buscopan compositium, (Boehringer Ingelheim) where necessary to relieve pain and intestinal spasm.

(6) Once antibiotic treatment has ceased, re-establishment of a beneficial intestinal flora can be aided by the use of live yoghurt, or probiotics or ground up fresh faecal pellets from an adult goat.

In ruminating animals antibiotic therapy may have deleterious effects on the rumen microflora.

Birth to 4 weeks

Dietary scour

(1) The majority of cases of diarrhoea in artificially reared kids between 2 and 12 weeks of age are related to nutrition; either directly, through sudden changes in concentration or type of milk replacer, changing between goat milk and milk replacer, overfeeding or varying the temperature at which the milk is fed, or indirectly through dirty utensils or contamination of feed. Correction of feeding practices and symptomatic treatment will result in the rapid resolution of uncomplicated nutritional diarrhoea but where secondary infection is involved the treatment may need to be more prolonged.

Nutritional scours may also predispose to, or coexist with bloat, colic and mesenteric torsion (see Chapter 15) all of which are potentially life threatening.

(2) In older kids and adults, overfeeding of concentrates without adequate roughage either through bad management or stealing food (see Chapters 14 and 15) will cause diarrhoea.

Similarly overgrazing on lush grass, excessive feeding of roots, e.g. mangolds, or kale, excess fruit or bread or mouldy hay will all cause digestive upsets.

E.coli

Coliform bacteria are commensals of the alimentary tract and can readily be identified on faecal culture. Enterotoxigenic *E.coli* (ETEC) are significant as a cause of diarrhoea in newborn kids and may complicate infections caused by cryptosporidia, rotavirus and coronavirus in kids up to 2–3 weeks of age. Other strains of *E.coli* cause septicaemia and chronic arthritis.

Aetiology

Enterotoxigenic *E.coli* produce an enterotoxin which causes the release of electrolytes and water from the cells lining the small intestine, resulting in diarrhoea. The enterotoxin is non-antigenic but ETEC have the antigenic K99 pilus which enables the bacterium to adhere to the intestinal epithelium.

Clinical signs

- Acute profuse, watery diarrhoea in very young kids.
- Dehydration and death.

Laboratory diagnosis

- Isolation of the organism on faecal culture.
- Detection of the K99 antigen by isolation on special media and slide testing for the antigen with specific antisera.
- Immunofluorescence of frozen sections of small intestine.

Treatment

- Antibiotics – orally or parenterally.
- General supportive therapy (qv).

Salmonellosis

Salmonellosis causes peracute septicaemia and sudden death in neonatal kids and an acute diarrhoea in kids and older goats, often following stress, and abortion in later gestation (see Chapter 2).
  Outbreaks of diarrhoea and abortion may occur concurrently.

Aetiology

- *S.typhimurium* and *S.dublin* are commonest but several other serotypes have been associated with disease.

Transmission

- Infection is most often acquired from other goats which are excreting the organism and are either clinical or preclinical cases of the disease or symptomless carriers. However, other sources of infection may occasionally be significant.
- Infection from food and water.
- Infection from other domestic animals or man.
- Infection from wild animals or birds.

Clinical signs:

- Lethargy.
- Diarrhoea, often profuse water and yellow ± dysentery.
- Abdominal pain.
- Dehydration.
- Death in severe cases.
- Sudden death in very young kids.

Postmortem findings

- Enteritis, abomasitis, septicaemia, enlarged mesenteric lymph nodes.

Laboratory diagnosis

- Culture of faeces – rectal swabs or faeces using selective media.
- Isolation of organism from mesenteric lymph nodes, hepatic lymph nodes, heart blood, spleen, lungs etc.
- The organism may be excreted in milk.

Treatment

- Antibiotics – orally or parenterally.
- General supportive therapy (qv).

Clostridium perfringens types B and C

Clostridium perfringens types B and C cause an acute haemorrhagic enteritis of kids under 3 weeks of age.

Aetiology

- Clostridia produce beta toxin in the small intestine causing local necrosis with resultant haemorrhagic diarrhoea.

Clincal signs

- Acute, profuse haemorrhagic diarrhoea.
- Abdominal pain.
- Death.

Postmortem findings

- Severe haemorrhagic enteritis affecting part or most of the ileum. The mucosa is congested and dark red and large deep ulcers are often present.

Laboratory investigation

Confirmation of the disease at postmortem is generally only possible in a freshly dead animal as beta toxin is very unstable.

- 20–30 ml of intestine contents to which 2–3 drops of chloroform have been added should be collected in a universal container and submitted to the laboratory.
- Gram stained impression smears from the small intestine show gram positive rods.
- Beta toxin can be demonstrated using mice protection tests with specific antisera or by an ELISA test.
- *Clostridium perfringens* is a normal inhabitant of the intestine and its isolation at postmortem is *not* necessarily significant.

Prevention

- Vaccination of the dam in late gestation to confer protection on the kids via the colostrum – see *Clostridium perfringens* type D in 'colic in kids'.

Treatment

- Administration of clostridial antitoxins (Lamb Dysentery antiserum – Coopers Pitman-Moore).

Campylobacter

Campylobacter spp. have occasionally been isolated from diarrhoeic kids and are a potential zoonotic hazard.

Viral diarrhoea

Rotavirus, Coronavirus and Adenovirus have been reported to cause diarrhoea in kids. Mixed infections with enterotoxigenic *E.coli* or *Cryptosporidia* may occur.

Rotavirus is the commonest enteric virus of goats.

Aetiology

- The virus infects and destroys the epithelial cells of villi in the small intestine, producing malabsorption and diarrhoea.

Clinical signs

- Acute, profuse watery diarrhoea, dehydration and death.
- Many kids will carry inapperent infections.

Laboratory investigation

- Demonstration of viral particles in faeces by electron microscopy.
- Demonstration of viral antigen in faeces by an ELISA test.
- Immunofluorescence on frozen intestinal section.

Other viruses such as a herpes virus have also been implicated in diarrhoea in goats but the clinical significance of these isolates is unclear.

Cryptosporidium

Aetiology

- *Cryptosporidium* spp. are small protozoan parasites related to enteric coccidia which parasitize the distal small intestine, caecum and colon, reducing the mucosal surface area resulting in malabsorption and deficiencies in mucosal enzymes, particularly lactose. The life cycle is direct and closely resembles that of other Eimerian coccidia, although it is as short as 3 or 4 days, so environmental contamination can reach high levels very rapidly.

Transmission

- *Cryptosporidium* lacks host specificity so one domestic species may spread infection to another.
- Purchased infected animals will introduce the disease into a herd.
- Mice and rats may act as a reservoir of infection.
- Infective oocysts are highly resistant and will persist in paddocks or in pens for over a year.
- Oocysts sporulate in the intestine and are immediately infective when passed in the faeces so rapid transmission occurs.
- Kids are usually infected within the first week of life and are fairly resistant by 4 weeks of age.

Clinical signs

- Watery diarrhoea in kids one to four weeks of age.
- Dehydration.
- Anorexia.
- High morbidity.
- Mortality may be high because of dehydration.

Postmortem examination

- Postmortem lesions resemble those due to other causes of diarrhoea.

Laboratory investigation

- Faecal smears air dried, fixed in methanol and stained with Giemsa will show the oocysts as blue circular structures with reddish granules.
- Oocysts can be concentrated by flotation in saturated salt or sugar solutions and examined by phase contrast microscopy or after staining.
- *Cryptosporidium* can be demonstrated in histological sections of small and large intestines provided the postmortem material is very fresh.

Treatment

- No specific therapy exists – anticoccidial drugs and antibiotics do not influence the course of the infections.
- Symptomatic treatment, including correction of dehydration (qv).

Prevention

- Once the disease is established on a premises, only steam or hot water cleaning of pens is likely to destroy the infective oocysts.

Strongyloides papillosus

Relatively common infection, occasionally producing diarrhoea in suckling kids. Kids are initially infected via the dam's milk so feeding of pooled milk or milk replacer will reduce the number of larvae transmitted. Subsequently infection is by ingestion or skin penetration and heavy infections may result in a localized dermatitis (see Chapter 10).

Diagnosis

- Faecal examination for typical embryonated eggs.

Treatment

- Any broad spectrum anthelmintics.

4–12 weeks

Gastrointestinal parasitism

Gastrointestinal parasitism is the major differential diagnosis in older kids or adult goats showing diarrhoea, unthriftiness, poor growth rates, anaemia or hypoproteinaemia.

Investigation of suspected gastrointestinal parasitism

(1) History.
(2) Clinical examination.
   Any of the following may indicate worm infestation, particularly in the kid or young goat, but all ages are potentially susceptible as only limited protective immune response develops with age.
   - reduced growth rate/weight loss (see Chapter 8)
   - reduced fibre growth
   - reduced milk production
   - diarrhoea
   - anaemia (see Chapter 17)
   - sudden death (see Chapter 18).

NB (a) Subclinical levels of infection may cause significant losses in production (weight gain, milk production etc) without other overt clinical signs. (b) Combinations of clinical signs may be seen as animals are usually parasitized by more than one species.

As in sheep, the main species involved in producing scouring are *Ostertagia* spp. and *Trichostrongylus* spp. *Haemonchus contortus* infection causes severe anaemia, oedema and lethargy.
Clinical signs and history may be diagnostic if not:

Laboratory diagnosis

Faecal egg counts

Kids – generally good correlation between egg counts, worm burden and disease:

   500–2000 eggs/g faeces = subclinical infection
   >2000   eggs/g faeces = clinical infection

1–2 weeks after treating with anthelmintics counts should approach zero. If not suspect anthelmintic resistance or drenching procedure.

Confusion may occur if kids are given anthelmintic treatment shortly before a faecal sample is taken as clinical signs may persist due to chronic intestinal damage even though egg counts are low.

Adults – correlation less exact and counts may be misleading.

(1) depressed egg production as a result of partial host immunity – worm burden and therefore damage greater than count suggests
(2) worm burden required to produce clinical disease depends on other factors such as nutrition and milk production level
(3) larvae may produce disease before egg production
(4) diurnal and seasonal variations in egg production occur.

NB Significant worm burdens can develop in deep litter systems given suitable conditions of temperature and humidity.

Postmortem examination

- Identify various worms present:
  Goats are infected with the same parasites that effect sheep and also some of the parasites that affect cattle:

  Abomasum: *Haemonchus contortus, Ostertagia* spp., *Trichostrongylus axei*

  Small intestine: *Trichostrongylus* spp., *Nematodirus* spp., *Bunostomum trigonocephalum, Cooperia curticei, Strongyloides papillosus*

  Large intestine: *Oesophagostomum columbianum, Chabertia ovina, Trichuris ovis*

- Estimate number of worms present: significance of numbers depends on other factors such as overall herd health, clinical signs etc.

  As a rough guide:

T. colubriformis	4000	= subclinical infection
	8000	= diarrhoea in young goats
	20 000	= death in young goats
H. contortus	500	= subclinical infection
	1000	= anaemia in young goats
	2500	= death in young goats

Plasma pepsinogen levels

Levels >3 i.u. may indicate severe ostertagiasis.

Haematology

Anaemia and hypoproteinaemia are consistent with *Haemonchosis and Trichostrongylosis.*

Treatment

- Only a limited number of anthelmintics have a product licence for goats.
- Drugs and dose rates of drugs for sheep cannot necessarily be directly related for use in goats (consult manufacturer if necessary). Higher dose rates often required in goats.
- Estimation of goats weight is difficult – easy to underdose.
- Milk withholding times important in dairy goats – not necessarily the same as for sheep or cattle (consult manufacturer). Any product not licensed for goats has a mandatory 7 day withholding time.
- Resistance of goat nematodes to benzimidazole anthelmintics has been reported in the UK.

Cross resistance occurs between all the benzimidozole and probenzimidozole anthelmentics.

No cross resistance occurs between benzimidozole group and levamisole or Ivermectin.

Cestode infection

Moniezia spp. commonly affect goats but clinical or subclinical disease has not been attributed to them. It is possible that if present in sufficient numbers the intestinal lumen could be occluded. Mebendazole and Febendazole are effective against tapeworms.

Coccidiosis

A major cause of diarrhoea, particularly in housed kids.

Aetiology

- Coccidia are protozoan parasites: goats are affected by 12 species of *Eimeria* which are all specific for the goat except *E. caprovina* which is transmissible between sheep and goats. Related protozoa such as *Isospora*, *Sarcocystis* and *Toxoplasma* do not generally multiply in the intestinal tract of the ruminant. The coccidial species of cattle, poultry or domestic pets do not cause coccidiosis in the goat.

Transmission

- All goats are infected with coccidia.
- It is probable that all kids are infected during their first few weeks of life and that management standards determine whether or not the levels of infection are sufficient to cause clinical signs of the disease. Kids become infected by ingestion of food, bedding and water contaminated with sporulated oocysts.
- Oocysts are ingested by the kid, rapidly undergo maturation and multiply. The cycling of a single oocyst could result in one to two million oocysts being passed 3–4 weeks later.
- Infection can occur indoors in intensive rearing situations or at pasture when the grass is sufficiently short for ingestion of oocysts lying on the soil surface.
- Oocysts are resistant to low temperature and will overwinter on pasture or indoors to provide a source of infection the following spring.

Epidemiology

- Kids become infected in the first few weeks of life with the highest incidence of clinical disease between 4 and 7 weeks of age. After this, faecal oocyst excretion decreases as the kids acquire immunity to coccidia.
- Stress factors such as weaning, transport, changes in diet and adverse weather conditions can also predispose to the development of clinical disease possibly by producing a relaxation of immunity.

Clinical signs

- Depression.
- Anorexia.
- Weight loss.
- Diarrhoea, possibly with blood and/or mucus.
- Dehydration.
- Death.

In severely infected kids massive release of meronts and merozoites from the intestinal cells can produce sudden onset colic, shock and collapse or kids may be found dead with no signs of diarrhoea.

Recovered kids may show illthrift with a reduced growth rate and poor fibre production.

Diagnosis

The diagnosis of clinical coccidiosis must be based on the history, observation of clinical signs, postmortem findings, faecal oocyst counts and oocyst speciation.

Diagnosis based on the number of oocysts in faecal samples poses a number of problems:

- All kids are infected with coccidia.
- A severe challenge and the subsequent asexual reproductions can result in considerable damage to the intestine and clinical signs in the prepatent phase before the sexual cycle occurs with release of oocysts in the faeces. In very heavy infections the damage to the intestinal mucosa may not leave enough epithelial cells in the villi for the sexual cycle to occur.
- The intestines may be so damaged by the infection that clinical signs, i.e. diarrhoea, persist after the peak of oocyst production.
- Normal kids may have 1000–1 000 000 oocysts/g faeces; clinically ill kids may have 100–10 000 000 oocysts/g faeces.
- Identification of the species of *Coccidia* present may be helpful.
- The predominant species in the faeces of the normal goat are *E.arloingi* and *E.hirci*. The most pathogenic species which predominate in kids which are clinically ill are *E. ninakohlyakimovae*, *E.caprina* and *E.christenseni*.

Postmortem findings

- Gross postmortem finds are often limited.
- Haemorrhagic or mucoid enteritis may be obvious in severe infections, but in less severe infections there is generally little haemorrhage into the intestine.
- Small white pinpoint lesions may be present on the mucosal surface of the intestine. Smears taken from these areas show the presence of meronts, gametocytes and oocysts.

Control

(1) *The environment*
- Avoid overcrowding.
  - Provide clean dry well strawed pens for each batch of kids.
- Do not mix kids of different age groups.
- Raise food and water containers above the floor to avoid faecal contamination.

- Slatted floors rather than deep litter may help reduce the oocyst level in some husbandry systems.

(2) The doe
- Feeding a coccidiostat to the does in late pregnancy will reduce oocyst output and thus contamination of the environment but enough oocysts will remain to infect the kids in intensive housing conditions and the coccidia can rapidly multiply in the non-immune kid.

(3) The kid
- Prophylatic medication may have some success in controlling coccidiosis by reducing the challenge to the kids and allowing them to develop immunity by exposure to a low number of oocysts. However, drug treatment in a contaminated environment will only have a temporary effect. Most drugs are coccidiostats with only a limited coccidiocidal effect.
- No anticoccidial drugs are specifically licensed for goats in the UK. Some, e.g. monsensin, have a narrow safety margin. Individual manufacturers should be contacted for their recommendations. The following have been used in small ruminants.
    (a) Sulphonamide compounds
        Sulphamethazine – 110 mg/kg body wt for 5 days every 3 weeks
        Sulphaquinoxalone – 8–70 mg/kg body wt for 5 days every 3 weeks
    (b) Amprolium – 5 mg/kg body weight for 21 days
    (c) Monensin – 1 mg/kg bodyweight
    (d) Salinomycin sodium
    (e) Decoquinate

Treatment
(1) Coccidiostats
    (a) Sulphadimidine tables and solutions
    (b) Sulphamethoxy pyridazine
    (c) Sulphapyrazole
    (d) Trimethoprim/sulphadiazine
    (e) Amprolium
    (f) Oral sulphonamide/antibiotic mixtures.
(2) Additional supportive therapy will be required in severe cases – fluids, intravenous corticosteroids or analgesics.

Helminthiasis may occur concurrently with coccidiosis.

Clostridium perfringens type D (entertoxaemia, pulpy kidney disease)

See Chapter 15.

Salmonella – (qv)

Giardiasis

Aetiology

- A protozoan parasite, *Giardia*.

Transmission

- Faecal contamination of water, food or environment by an infected animal.

Clinical signs

- Chronic but sometimes intermittent watery diarrhoea.

Laboratory investigation

- Demonstration of motile flagellates in wet faecal smears stained with Giemsa to show the flagellae, pear shaped central bodies and binucleate appearance.
- Cysts can be concentrated by flotation in zinc sulphate.

Treatment

- Giardia infection is readily susceptible to metronidazole (Flagyl, RMB) while being unsusceptible to routine antibiotic therapy.

Public health considerations

- Giardia is a possible zoonosis by direct contact with sick animals or through faecal contamination.

Nutritional factors – (qv)

Campylobacter jejuni – (qv)

Toxic agents causing diarrhoea

Poisonous plants

May be eaten direct or in hay – plants reported to cause diarrhoea include aconite, bluebell, box, buckthorn, dog's mercury, irises, rhododendron, spurges and wild arum.

Mycotoxins

Fungal toxins in mouldy conserved fodder or badly dried cereals.

Poisonous minerals

- Copper (footbaths, sprays etc); – see Chapter 14.
- Basic slag, nitrogenous or other types of *fertilizer* from recently top dressed pasture.
- Industrial waste – fluorides, arsenicals, barium, chromium, mercury, zinc and selenium.
- Fruit sprays.
- Teart pastures – molybdenum.
- Lead – access to old paint or batteries – (qv).

Drugs

Sulphonamides, carbon tetrachloride, copper sulphate, warfarin etc.

Over 12 weeks

- Parasitic gastoenteritis – (qv).
- Coccidiosis – (qv).
- *Cl. perfringens* type D – see Chapter 15.
- Salmonella – (qv).
- Nutritional factors – (qv).
- Toxic agents – (qv).
- Liver disease – see Chapter 14.
  Hepatic disease and bile duct obstruction leads to a decrease in the level of bile salts in the alimentary tract. This together with general liver distension causes gastrointestinal disturbances of anorexia and constipation, with attacks of diarrhoea.
- Copper deficiency – see Chapter 5.
  Results in anaemia, illthrift, poor coat, infertility and diarrhoea in growing and adult goats.
- *Johne's disease* – see Chapter 8.
  Diarrhoea is an uncommon finding in Johne's disease in goats but may occur terminally.

Further reading

General

Blackwell, R. E. (1983) Enteritis and diarrhoea. *Vet. Clin. North Amer.: Large Animal Practice*, **5** (3), November 1983, 557–570
Thompson, K. G. (1985) Enteric diseases of goats. *Proc. Course in Goat Husbandry and Medicine, Massey University*, November 1985, 78–85

Helminthiasis

Baldock, C. (1984) Helminthiasis in goats. *Proc. Univ. Sydney Post Grad Comm. Vet. Sci.*, **73**, 450–467
Lloyd, S. (1982) Control of parasites in goats. *Goat Vet. Soc. J.*, **3** (1), 2–6
Lloyd, S. (1987) Endoparasitic disease in goats. *Goat Vet. Soc. J.*, **8** (1), 32–39

Coccidiosis

Gregory, M. and Norton, C. (1986) Anticoccidials. *In Practice*, January 1986, 33–35
Gregory, M. and Norton, C. (1986) Caprine coccidiosis. *Goat Vet. Soc. J.*, **7** (2), 32–34
Howe, P. A. (1984) Coccidiosis. *Proc. Univ. Sydney Post Grad. Comm. Vet. Sci.*, **73**, 468–472
Lloyd, S. (1987) Endoparasitic disease in goats. *Goat Vet. Soc. J.*, **8** (1), 32–39
Van Veen, T. W. S. (1986) Coccidiosis in ruminants. *Comp. Cont. Ed. Pract. Vet.*, **8** (10), F52–F58

Cryptosporidiosis/giardiasis

Angus, K. W. (1987) Cryptosporidiosis in domestic animals and humans. *In Practice*, March 1987, 47–49
Kirkpatrick, C. E. (1989) Giardiasis in large animals. *Comp. Cont. Ed. Pract. Vet.*, **II** (1), 80–84
Lloyd, S. (1986) Parasitic zoonoses. *Goat Vet. Soc. J.*, **7** (2), 39–44

14 Colic in adult goats

Initial assessment
Diarrhoea/enteritis
Indigestion (ruminal atony)
Acute impaction of the rumen (acidosis)
Ruminal tympany
Secondary ruminal tympany ('choke')
Enterotoxaemia
Left-sided displacement of the abomasum
Urolithiasis
Liver disease
Toxic minerals
Fertilizer ingestion
Post kidding problems
Plant poisoning

Diarrhoea/enteritis
Indigestion (ruminal atony)
Acidosis (ruminal impaction)
Ruminal tympany
   primary (frothy bloat)
   secondary (choke)
Enterotoxaemia (*Clostridium perfringens* type D)
Abomasal ulceration
Left-sided displacement of the abomasum
Urolithiasis
Liver disease
Toxic minerals, e.g. copper, lead
Fertilizer ingestion
Post kidding problems
   Metritis
   Retained kid
Cystitis
Plant poisoning

Initial assessment

- The feeding history – overfeeding, change in diet, mouldy feed etc.
- General physical examination – to determine whether the problem is related to a specific alimentary condition, associated with a more general disease, or not connected with the alimentary tract at all (e.g. urolithiasis).
- Specific examination of the digestive system
  Visual inspection – abdominal contour from behind, abdominal distension
  Palpation of the left abdominal wall and rumen – filling of the rumen
  Percussion – tympanitic sounds, pain
  Auscultation – rumen mobility, sounds of left-sided abomasal displacement.

Further investigations

- Passage of a stomach tube allows release of accumulated gas and the collection of a sample of ruminal fluid. A simple gag to facilitate stomach tubing can be made by drilling a hole in a piece of wood.
- Trocharization of the left paralumber fossa releases accumulated gas.

Examination of rumen contents

- Measure pH with indicater papers, pH 4.5–5.0 suggests a moderate degree of abnormality. A pH <4.5 suggests severe rumen acidosis and requires emergency treatment.
- Methylene blue reduction test measures the redox potential of the ruminal fluid and reflects the level of activity of aerobic rumen microflora; 20 ml of ruminal fluid is added to 1 ml of 0.03% methylene blue solution in a test tube and the time required for the methylene blue to decolorize is measured. The faster the decolorization the more active the microflora – microfloral inactivity will give results of 15 minutes or longer and severe rumen acidosis >5 minutes. A normal goat with a high concentrate ration will have a time of 1–3 minutes and a goat on an all hay diet 3–6 minutes.

Diarrhoea/enteritis

See Chapter 13.

Indigestion (ruminal atony)

Aetiology

- Minor degrees of dietary mismanagement, particularly inadequate protein and energy with a high fibre diet, mouldy or frosted feeds, a moderate overfeeding of concentrates or insufficient water, produce various degrees of ruminal impaction and atony.
- Oral dosing with antibiotics or sulphonamides (due to destruction of the normal ruminal flora).
- Lack of exercise.
- Oral dosing with linseed oil produces a foul tasting cud which is often spat out and normal chewing of the cud ceases.

Clinical findings

- Reduced appetite or complete anorexia.
- Reduced milk yield.
- Constipation with small amounts of faeces or occasionally diarrhoea.
- Generally a firm, pliable rumen palpable on the left side but occasionally moderate degrees of tympany as ruminal atony becomes established.

- No signs or only weak signs of rumination.
- Often few signs of abdominal pain, although occasionally typical spasmodic colic signs such as pawing the ground with the front feet, looking at the abdomen, frequent getting up and down and grinding of teeth.

Treatment

- Many mildly affected animals will recover spontaneously. In other cases, symptomatic treatment should be adopted.
- Use Epsom Salts (200 g) in 300 ml water as a drench on the first day, then 100 g, 75 g and 50 g on successive days if necessary.
- Give vegetable oil (30 ml) in about 100 ml liquid paraffin as a drench.
- Rehydration if necessary.
- Relief of pain where present.
- In animals with a recurrent problem, *bran mashes* two or three times weekly may help prevent impaction – mix four handfuls of bran scalded with sufficient boiling water to make a crumbly mash and leave to stand for 10 minutes.
- Feed on browsings, leaves and branches, to encourage the resumption of cudding.
- Re-establish ruminal microflora with yoghurt, probiotics or by drenching fresh rumen contents or ground up faeces.

NB Abomasal impaction may occur in animals with poor rumination. The abomasum is palpable in the low right abdomen. Treat as for ruminal atony.

Acute impaction of the rumen (acidosis)

Aetiology

- Excess ingestion of high energy feeds such as barley, wheat, dairy cake etc. results in a rapid fermentation of the carbohydrate in the feed with the formation of large quantities of lactic acid decreasng the rumen pH. As the pH falls, rumen motility decreases and the normal rumen microflora are destroyed and replaced by lactobacilli and streptococci. The lactic acid produces a severe rumenitis with necrosis of the mucous membrane and lactic acid and the toxic products from the degeneration of the rumen bacteria are absorbed causing a toxaemia. The ruminal contents are hypertonic to plasma, so fluids are lost into the alimentary tract resulting in diarrhoea and dehydration.

- Certain feeds which are acidic in their own right, e.g. mangolds, apples, rhubarb, etc., may produce acidosis if they are suddenly fed in large quantities.
- Secondary infection by fungi or bacteria such as *Fusibacterium necrophorum* may lead to a more prolonged rumenitis after the animal has survived the acute disease.

Clinical signs

- Lethargy.
- Anorexia.
- Abdominal pain – grinding of teeth, kicking at abdomen.
- Subnormal temperature.
- Fast, weak pulse.
- Ruminal movements absent.
- Diarrhoea.
- Death.
- Laminitis (see Chapter 6) may develop in animals which have recovered due to changes in the corium of the feet.

Treatment

- Mild cases can be treated as for indigestion (qv).
- Drenching with 100 g sodium bicarbonate will help reduce the acidosis (but overdosing may lead to alkalosis); alternatively 15 ml milk of magnesia is a good antacid that will not convert to metabolic alkalosis if excess is given. Repeat in 3–4 hours if necessary.
- Oral antibiotics, e.g. tetracyclines may help restrict the growth of the lactic acid producing bacteria.
- Dehydration should be corrected with parenteral administration of 1–2 litres of isotonic fluids together with sodium bicarbonate.
- B vitamins, particularly thiamine will aid detoxification.
- Surgical – rumenotomy should be performed in serious cases, the rumen completely emptied and washed out and the contents replaced by hay, water and preferably rumen contents from a normal goat.
- The re-establishment of the normal rumenal microflora should be assisted by dosing with yoghurt, probiotics, ground up faecal pellets etc.

Ruminal tympany

Ruminal tympany should be distinguished from other causes of abdominal distension (Table 14.1).

Table 14.1 Abdominal distension in adult goats

Ruminal tympany	
Pregnancy	
Hydrometra	— see Chapter 1
Ascites	— uncommon in goats may arise in fascioliasis as a result of blood loss and decreased hepatic synthesis of albumin and occasionally from chronic liver congestion or cardiac failure
Abdominal fat	— goats carry their fat deposits intra-abdominally rather than subcutaneously
Dropped stomach	— in British Toggenburgs, the abdominal muscles may drop ventrolaterally in late pregnancy so that the abdomen subsequently remains lower than normal
Ventral hernia	

Primary ruminal tympany (frothy bloat)

Aetiology

- Grazing lush pastures, particularly clover or lucerne in the spring; sudden introduction of grass clippings or excessive vegetable waste etc. produces a rumen filled with gas or frothy material.

Clinical signs

- Depression.
- Abdominal pain – teeth grinding, shifting of weight on the feet, kicking at the abdomen.
- Abdominal distension – more obvious in the left flank but the whole of the abdomen is enlarged.
- Dyspnoea – mouth breathing, extension of the head, protrusion of the tongue.

Treatment

(1) *First aid treatment by owner*
  - Drench with 50 to 100 ml of any non-toxic vegetable or mineral oil or with a proprietary bloat drench; or with

8–10 ml of medical turpentine in 100 ml liquid paraffin. In an emergency 10 ml of washing up liquid will suffice. Massage the abdomen to spread the oil.

- Stand the goat with the front feet raised, tie a 30 cm stick through the mouth like a bridle and smear honey or treacle on the back of the tongue to promote continual chewing. Gentle exercise may encourage eructation.
- Trocharize the rumen on the left side with a 14 or 16 g 38 mm or 50 mm needle.

(2) Veterinary treatment continues the treatment started by the owner with release of gas by means of a stomach tube or trocharization with a needle or sheep trocar and cannula. Oil or bloat remedy can be introduced directly into the rumen through a cannula.
- Increase the fibre in the diet by feeding hay before a return to feeding legumes or grazing.

Prevention

- Allow only limited access to grazing.
- Avoid any sudden introduction of fermentable material to the diet.
- Provide sufficient fibre in the diet in the form of hay.
- Smearing vegetable oil on the coat before grazing will promote a regular intake of oil by licking so preventing gas build up.

Secondary ruminal tympany ('choke')

Aetiology

- A physical obstruction to eructation causes a build up of gas in the rumen, e.g. *oesophageal obstruction* caused by a foreign body such as a piece of apple or rootcrop or a tumour at the region of thoracic inlet.
- Spasm of the reticuloruminal musculature in *tetanus* and interference with oesophageal groove functions in cases of *diaphragmatic hernia* may also lead to chronic ruminal tympany.
- A degree of ruminal tympany may be observed in diseases such as *listeriosis* because of pharyngeal paralysis.

Treatment

- First aid treatment by the owner as for primary tympany – small amounts of oil may help lubricate an obstruction.
- Veterinary treatment – trocharization to relieve the build up of gas.
- Administration of an antispasmolytic drug such as Buscopan compositum (Boehringer Ingelheim) to aid relaxation of oesophageal musculature around a foreign body.
- Consider oesophagostomy where the foreign body is palpable in the neck if conservative methods are unsuccessful.

Enterotoxaemia (*Clostridium perfringens* type D pulpy kidney disease)

Enterotoxaemia is a potential problem in all ages of goat as the causative agent is present in most herds (see Chapter 15).

Abomasal ulceration

Aetiology

- Poorly documented but probably due to a high concentrate/low roughage diet, particularly in early lactation. Ulceration may be a sequel to chronic acidosis and rumen stasis.

Clinical signs

- Many goats with superficial abomasal ulceration show no apparent illness or only occasionally become inappetent. However, deeper ulceration will lead to more severe clinical signs.
- Changes in the abomasal tone and motility will in turn affect the motility of the rumen and reticulum.
- Perforation with omental adhesion which seals the perforation produces low grade intermittent pain, with grinding of teeth, intermittent pyrexia, reduced ruminoreticular movement, weight loss, reduced milk yield, marked inappetence and intermittent diarrhoea.
- Perforation without the defect being sealed may result in an acute diffuse peritonitis and death.
- Severe haemorrhage may occur and produce displacement (see below) with adhesions to the left side of the abdomen.

Treatment

- Symptomatic; correct the diet.
- Metaclopramide (Emequell, Smith Kline Beecham) 0.5–1.0 mg/kg i.v. then i.m. every 12–24 hours as necessary to restore abomasal tone and encourage emptying.
- Broad spectrum antibiotics.

Left-sided displacement of the abomasum

Aetiology

- Left-sided displacement of the abomasum is poorly documented in the goat, but is probably related to high levels of concentrate feeding in late pregnancy. During pregnancy the abomasum is pushed under the rumen by the expanding uterus. After parturition the rumen resumes its normal position trapping the abomasum.

Clinical signs

- Selective anorexia – refuse concentrates but eat hay.
- Reduced ruminal contractions; rarely cud.
- Initial constipation, then diarrhoea.
- Secondary ketosis – smell of ketones on breath, positive Rothera's reaction on milk.
- Auscultation of the left flank reveals abnormal sounds – high pitched metallic tinkling and ringing sounds which may be spontaneous or can be elicited.

Treatment

- A spontaneous cure may occur with exercise and access to browsings.
- Conservative treatment with starvation and rolling.
- Surgical replacement and anchorage.
- After spontaneous cure or surgery, concentrate feeding should be reintroduced very gradually over a period of two or three weeks.

Urolithiasis

- Metabolic disease of male goats, particularly castrates of any age and male kids but occasionally entire males of any age, characterized by the formation of calculi within the urinary tract and urethral blockage.

- The calculi are generally phosphatic but oxalates and silicates sometimes occur.
- In the UK, urolithiasis is virtually always associated with concentrate feeding.

Aetiology

(1) Anatomy
- Male animals affected; female can pass calculi easily through their shorter, wider urethra.
- Castration arrests penile development so the urethra remains narrow.
- Mature animals have a larger urethra than immature animals. *Young castrated animals are at greatest risk.*

(2) Urinary phosphorus excretion
- High levels of urinary phosphorus increase the likelihood of the formation of insoluble phosphates and urinary calculi.
- Factors which increase urinary phosphorus excretion predispose to calculi formation.
- Urinary phosphorus excretion is normally very low in ruminants as any excess phosphorus absorbed is secreted back into the digestive system via the saliva and excreted in the faeces. However, a number of factors may lead to increased urinary phosphorus:

   (a) *High levels of dietary phosphorus* – at a certain level the salivary phosphorus recycling system becomes saturated and urinary phosphorus excretion occurs.
   (b) *Low levels of dietary calcium (low calcium:phosphorus ratio)* – a high calcium:phosphorus ratio in the diet reduces the incidence of calculi formation by decreasing the absorption of phosphorus from the gut, thus reducing urinary phosphate levels. Conversely rations low in calcium increase phosphorus intake.
   (c) *Low fibre diet* – goats on high grain/low fibre diets secrete much lower amounts of saliva than animals on high roughage diets thus decreasing the amount of phosphorus excreted in the faeces.
   (d) *Low urine output* – any reduction in voluntary water intake will lead to decreased urine volume and increase the likelihood of calculi formation. Feeding

concentrates instead of roughages significantly reduces the urine volume.

  (e) *Dietary magnesium levels* – some research has suggested that high magnesium levels *per se* do not cause urolithiasis and may in fact reduce the incidence of calculi formation by reducing urinary phosphorus excretion.

  (f) *Genotypic predisposition* – in sheep, individual differences in phosphorus metabolism have been shown to have a genetic basis – phosphorus is excreted mainly in the faeces by some sheep and in the urine by others. It is probable that there is a similar situation in goats – a familial tendency to calculi formation has been shown in Saanen males.

    There are definite breed differences in sheep – it is not known if the same applies to goats.

  (g) *Alkaline urine pH* – phosphate calculi form more readily in alkaline urine.

(3) Oxalate containing plants
- Calcium oxalate crystals may form in animals fed on oxalate containing plants such as sugar beet tops.
- This has led to a widespread misconception among goatkeepers that sugar beet *pulp* should not be fed to male goats – there is no scientific evidence to support this theory.

Clinical signs

- Anorexia, lethargy.
- Signs of abdominal pain – grinding of teeth, looking at abdomen, kicking at abdomen.
- Reluctant to walk; stands with legs stretched out.
- Strains to urinate; may dribble urine before complete blockage occurs; small calculi may collect on preputial hairs.
- Palpation of the abdomen is resented; tight bladder may be palpable in kids.
- Rupture of the urethra results in infiltration of urine into the perineal subcutaneous tissues, bladder rupture results in urine accumulation in the scrotum or intra-abdominally.

Diagnosis

- Clinical signs.

NB Initial signs may be mild, i.e. lethargy, inappetence, slight straining – careful examination may be required over one or two hours.

- Examination of the urethral process, palpation of urethra. Angoras can be sat on their rump or laid on their back with front and back legs tied tightly together so that the penis can be exteriorized and held with a swab or cotton wool; larger dairy goats will require sedation with Xylazine.
- Radiography will help locate calculi and determine numbers of calculi present.

Treatment

- The penis should be exteriorized (see diagnosis) and the urethral process examined – this is the commonest site of blockage. Sedation with Xylazine may provide sufficient muscle relaxation to allow a stone to be passed. In most cases, the urethral process will require removing with scissors. If only the urethral process is blocked, urine flow will occur within 5 minutes.
- Complete catheterization to the bladder is anatomically impossible – catheters will not pass the ischial arch as they enter a diverticulum of the urethra – but retrograde catheterization from the bladder to the penis is possible following surgery.
- Where further stones are present or the blockage is not at the urethral process, a urethrostomy will be necessary to locate and remove the obstruction. Radiography will help locate the calculi.
- In castrates, a permanent urethrostomy opening is made, but owners should be warned of problems with premature closing of the orifice and the backward direction of urination (important in driving goats).
- Stud males are difficult to treat as any surgery must not impair fertility. Occasionally a single calculi can be palpated and removed and the urethra sutured once the potency of the distal urethra has been established. Bladder stones can be removed at cystotomy and individual urethral stones removed. However, most affected stud males are destroyed.

General management for all male goats

(1) Ensure adequate water intake
   - clean water should always be available – change twice daily

- give warm water in cold weather
- check the height and suitability of any automatic drinkers and check that the goats know how to use them.

(2) Feed palatable fodder – *good* hay, pea straw etc.

(3) Feed dried grass products, e.g. lucerne, instead of concentrates – lucerne has the added advantage of being high in calcium.

(4) Do not feed buffers, e.g. $NaHCO_3$.

(5) Feed a well balanced diet with 2:1 Ca:P ration.
- Add calcium as calcium chloride to adjust ration where necessary.

(6) Do not add P to concentrate diets.

Additional control measures in problem herds/flocks

Control

- Control in the UK is generally directed towards prevention of phosphatic calculi forming; but it is sensible to have the calculi analysed after each episode and to measure the urine pH before beginning control measures.
- Increase the salt (NaCl) content of the ration – an increase to 4% will be required to alter water intake. Up to 9% NaCl can be fed before decreasing palatability.
- Add urine pH modifiers, e.g. NH_4 Cl (2% of concentrate ration), fishmeal, citrus pulp, maize gluten.
- Give NH_4 Cl by mouth – 15 g in water daily.

Liver disease

A general increase in the size of the liver or specific parenchymal changes may result in abdominal pain, either a localized pain detectable by palpation or more generalized pain with changes in posture and unwillingness to move. Other clinical signs of liver disease include: oedema, ascites, hepatic encephalopathy (see Chapter 11), photosensitivity (see Chapter 10), anorexia, constipation, diarrhoea (see Chapter 13), jaundice (qv), or weight loss (see Chapter 8).

Diagnosis

- *Biochemistry* – AsT, GGT, GLDH, SDH, albumin, globulin; serum protein electrophoresis.

The biochemical profile shows whether there is significant liver disease and gives some indication of the type of liver pathology present.

(a) *Primary hepatocellular disease*
Damage to hepatocytes gives an increase in serum of specific hepatocyte enzymes. In goats these are glutamate dehydrogenase (GLDH) and sorbitol dehydrogenase (SDH). In the absence of damage to the bile duct system, gamma glutamyltransferase (GGT) remains low.

(i)   Severe anaemia – haemorrhage, haemolytic disease, haemonchosis
(ii) Copper poisoning (qv)
(iii) Shock
(iv) Congestive cardiac failure
(v)   Bacteraemia – liver abscess, Salmonellosis

(b)   *Cholangiohepatitis*
Damage to the biliary system and the hepatocytes results in elevated serum GLDH *and* GGT.
(i)   Fascioliasis (qv)
(ii) Bacterial cholangitis
(iii) Pyrrolizidine alkaloid poisoning (qv)
(iv) Primary neoplasia
(v)   Metastatic neoplasia
(vi) Aflatoxicosis

(c)   *Hepatic cirrhosis*
Persistent liver damage and fibrosis from whatever cause results in a decrease in the functional liver mass. Early or moderate fibrosis is difficult to detect biochemically but when severe will result in decreased serum albumin and increased globulin; GGT and GLDH may be moderately elevated.

NB Jaundice is an uncommon sign in the goat even with severe hepatocellular damage but may occur

• in haemolytic disease where there is excess production of bilirubin, e.g. copper toxicity, leptospirosis, eperythrozoonosis and poisoning by Brassicas or onions.
• following bile duct obstruction, e.g. fascioliasis.

With haemolytic disease, most of the bilirubin is indirect as it has not been conjugated by the hepatocytes; in cholestatic diseases more of the bilirubin will be direct.
Urine bilirubin may not be elevated in haemolytic disease

because unconjugated bilirubin is bound to serum protein and will not be filtered by the kidney. Conjugated bilirubin in obstructive cholestasis is water soluble and may be detected in urine.

Urine urobilinogen may be increased in haemolytic jaundice because of increased production but is absent in obstructive cholestasis because no bilirubin is converted into urobilinogen in the intestine.

Liver biopsy

Use a transthoracic approach via the right 9th intercostal space.

(a) Primary hepatocellar disease – necrosis of hepatocytes, cirrhosis, fatty changes, biliary hyperplasia.
(b) Bile duct obstruction – plugs of bile in canaliculi, biliary cirrhosis etc.

Toxic minerals

Copper poisoning

Goats are relatively more resistant to copper poisoning than sheep but poisoning may occur from high copper mineral licks, eating pig rations containing high levels of copper, drinking footbaths or dosing with copper sulphate. Calf milk replacers containing high copper levels have also been implicated. Low dietary levels of zinc and molybdenum, which are copper antagonists, may increase copper intake even when dietary copper levels are not obviously high. Copper accumulates in the liver until maximum hepatic levels are reached when copper is released into the blood stream causing an acute intravascular haemolysis.

Clinical signs
- Often sudden death.
- Dull, lethargic, pyrexic.
- Severe abdominal pain.
- Mucoid diarrhoea.
- Haemoglobinuria/anaemia if goat survives long enough.
- Jaundice.

Laboratory findings
- Heinz body anaemia
- Elevated liver euzyme
- Marked bilirubinaemia

Postmortem findings

- Liver enlarged, friable, icteric.
- Entire carcase may be jaundiced.
- Kidneys dark green/black

Diagnosis

- Liver, kidney and faecal copper levels markedly elevated.

Treatment

- Ammonium tetrathiomolybdate either i.v./1.7 mg/kg or s.c. 3.4 mg/kg bodyweight in 3 doses on alternate days.

Lead poisoning

See Chapter 11.

Fertilizer ingestion

See Chapter 13.

Post kidding problems

Metritis

See Chapter 4.

Retained kid

See Chapter 4.

Cystitis

Cystitis occurs sporadically, particularly in does. Some does will merely show frequent urination with small amounts of urine being passed but acute cases will show moderate abdominal pain and occasionally systemic illness.

NB (1) Many does will urinate frequently when nervous; (2) It is sometimes difficult to distinguish between the end result of hydrometra (see Chapter 1), i.e. 'cloudburst' and cystitis. In most cloudbursts the fluid is rapidly released with sudden decrease in abdominal size and wetting of flanks and perineum but occasionally the fluid is released slowly over a few days with intermittent straining and passing of small amounts of fluid.

Plant poisoning

See Chapter 20.

Further reading

Urolithiasis

Baxendell, S. A. (1984) Urethral calculi in goats. *Proc. Univ. Sydney Post. Grad. Comm. Vet. Sci.*, **73**, 495–497
Cuddeford, D. (1988) Ruminant urolithiasis: cause and prevention. *Goat Vet. Soc. J.*, **10** (1), 10–14
Oehme, F. W. and Tillman, H. (1965) Diagnosis and treatment of ruminal urolithiasis. *JAVMA*, **147**, 1331–1339

Liver disease

Ellinson, R. S. (1985) Some aspects of clinical pathology in goats. *Proc. Course in Goat Husbandry and Medicine, Massey University*, November 1985, 105–122
Pearson, E. G. (1981) Differential diagnosis of icterus in large animals. *Calif. Vet.*, **2**, 25–31
Pearson, E. G. and Craig, A. M. (1980) The diagnosis of liver disease in equine and food animals. *Mod. Vet. Pract.*, **61** (3), 233–237

Acute impaction of the rumen

Michell, R. (1990) Ruminant acidosis. *In Practice*, November 1990, 245–249

15 Colic in kids

Diarrhoea
Abomasal bloat
Mesenteric torsion
Coccidiosis
Ruminal bloat
Constipation
Clostridium perfringens type D
Urolithiasis
Visceral cysticercosis
Plant poisoning

See also Chapter 14 – Colic in adult goats.

Any colic signs in kids should be treated as a potential emergency and the owner encouraged to seek veterinary help if the signs persist. Kids regularly die after quite short periods of abdominal pain.

- Diarrhoea/enteritis.
- Abomasal bloat.
- Mesenteric torsion.
- Coccidiosis.
- Ruminal bloat.
- Constipation.
- Enterotoxaemia (*Clostridium perfringens* type D).
- Urolithiasis.
- Visceral cysticercosis.
- Plant poisoning.

Diarrhoea

See Chapter 13.

Abomasal bloat

Abomasal bloat is common in artificially reared kids and is a significant cause of death in kids between 4 and 12 weeks of age. It should be distinguished from other causes of abdominal distension (Table 15.1).

Table 15.1 Abdominal distension in kids

(1) Birth to 1 week	
Prematurity	— see Chapter 5
Congenital abnormalities	— alimentary defect, e.g. imperforate anus cardiac or kidney defect (ascites)
High alimentary obstruction	— pyloric stenosis or obstruction, abomasal torsion
(2) Older kids	
Abomasal bloat	
Ruminal bloat	
Mesenteric torsion (intestinal bloat)	
'Pot belly'	— inadequate nutrition parasitism

Aetiology

- Poorly understood, but probably related to the rapid ingestion of large quantities of milk, leading to excessive fermentation and rapid distension of the abdomen with gas and fluid.

Clinical signs

- Abdominal distension with drum like tension on left and right sides.
- Colicky pain – grinding of teeth, yawning, constant stretching of the back.
- Diarrhoea.
- Shock.
- Death.

The condition may present as a 'sudden death' (Chapter 18) with the kid being found dead in the morning. All cases of bloat even if mild should be treated seriously and the kid checked at regular intervals.

Treatment

- Mild cases may respond to administration of a drench of a tablespoonful of vegetable oil or a proprietary bloat drench. Linseed oil is recommended in many older goat books but is not suitable as a drench as it may cause cessation of rumination since the regurgitation of stomach contents containing the oil is offensive in the mouth.

  More severe cases will require veterinary attention:

- Release pressure by trocharizing the abdomen on the left side with a 16 or 18 g needle.
- Give Buscopan Compositum (Boehringer Ingelheim) either intravenously or intramuscularly to relieve spasm and pain.
- Metaclopramide (Emequell, Smith Kline Beecham) 0.5–1.0 mg/kg i.v. may help restore abomasal tone and promote emptying.
- Administer broad spectrum antibiotics intramuscularly or intravenously.
- Fluid therapy for shocked kid.

Prevention

- Regular feeding with milk at the correct temperature and concentration.

- Consider feeding whole goat milk in problem herds – but this is more expensive and there is the danger of CAE spread.
- Kids fed from bowls rather than bottles are possibly more prone to bloat (due to more rapid intake of milk?) – consider bottle feeding or a multisuckling system in these herds, but this is more time consuming.
- Early wean any kid which has repeat episodes of bloat.

Mesenteric torsion

Mesenteric torsion leads to infarction of the abomasum, intestine or caecum.

Aetiology

- The aetiology of the condition is poorly understood but it occurs most commonly in artificially reared kids, probably after an excessive feed of milk in a short time. Torsions occasionally occur in older animals but the predisposing factors in these cases are not known.

Clinical findings

- As for bloat with severe abdominal pain distended abdomen and intermittent piercing screams; the kid may throw itself about.
- Kids are often found dead.
- Torsion should be considered in cases of bloat that do not respond to treatment.

Postmortem findings

- The affected portion of the alimentary tract is enlarged, dark red and filled with gas or blood-stained fluid.
- Careful examination reveals a twist in the mesentery.

Treatment

- Surgical intervention to correct the torsion may be effective if the condition is diagnosed early. Supportive therapy with intravenous fluids is essential to combat shock, together with analgesics such as flunixin meglamine (Finadyne, Schering Plough).

NB Other abdominal catastrophes such as intussusception will also produce signs of severe colic.

Coccidiosis

Intense colic and shock can be produced by the damage to the intestinal cells during release of meronts and merozoites so that kids may be found collapsed or dead.

Ruminal bloat

Rumen bloat may occur in kids during weaning.

Aetiology

- Sudden dilation of the abomasum by rapid intake of milk causes inhibition of forestomach motility.
- Failure of the oesophageal groove closure reflex allows milk to leak into rumen leading to excessive fermentation.
- Secondary to ruminal stasis and/or diarrhoea.
- Secondary to oesophageal obstruction (choke).

Clinical signs and *treatment* are as for abomasal bloat.

Prevention

- Correct feeding technique – establish a routine to ensure oesophageal groove closure at feeding; smaller feeds more frequently.
- If the bloat is repetitive wean the kid completely as early as possible.

Constipation

Constipation seems to be quite common in artificially reared kids in certain herds presumably as a result of management practices.

Aetiology

- Excess of concentrates with insufficient water intake?, as a sequel to *abomasal impaction*?

Clincal signs

- Depressed.
- Frequent unsuccessful attempts to defaecate.
- Low grade abdominal pain – stretching, yawning.
- Unwilling to feed or take milk.

Treatment

- Drench with a tablespoonful (15 ml) of liquid paraffin with about 2 teaspoonfuls (10 ml) of vegetable oil or proprietary colic drench containing turpentine oil and polymethylisoloxone (Gaseous Fluid, Day Son & Hewitt).

Clostridium perfringens type D (enterotoxaemia, pulpy kidney disease)

Aetiology

- *Clostridium perfringens* type D produces epsilon toxin in the small intestine. Rapid proliferation of the organism in response to dietary changes such as overgrowing lush pasture or overfeeding cereals results in toxin being absorbed into the bloodstream and damage to blood vessels in the brain, lungs and heart.

Transmission

- *Cl. perfringens* is present in the intestine of normal sheep and goats and has also been isolated from soil.

Clinical signs

- Peracute – sudden death or terminal shocked condition with convulsions.
- Acute
  diarrhoea, initially yellow green and soft later watery with mucous, blood and shreads of intestinal mucosa
  sternal and later lateral recumbency
  severe abdominal pain – pitiful intermittent cry of pain
  shock – cold extremities
  paddling movements and throwing back of head prior to death.

A chronic form has been described in adult goats showing periodic bouts of severe diarrhoea and wasting which responds to vaccination.

Postmortem findings

- Pericardial fluid that clots on exposure to air.
- Petechial or ecchymotic haemorrhages on the epicardium, endocardium, diaphragm, small intestine serosa and abdominal muscles.

- Mucosa of small intestine inflamed.
- 'Pulpy kidneys' may or may not be present.
- Symmetrical areas of haemorrhage, oedema and liquefaction in the brain, particularly the basal ganglia, focal symmetrical encephalomalacia (see Chapter 11).

Laboratory investigation

- Confirmation of the disease even at postmortem is generally difficult and only possible in a freshly dead animal.
- Twenty to thirty ml of intestine contents to which 2–3 drops of chloroform have been added should be collected in a universal container and submitted to the laboratory.
- *Cl. perfringens* type D is a normal inhabitant of the gut and may be found, with its toxin, in healthy animals.
- Gram stained impression smears from the small intestine show gram positive rods.
- Epsilon toxin can be demonstrated using mice protection tests with specific antisera or by an ELISA test.
- Urine collected from the bladder may contain glucose.

Treatment

- Administration of *Cl. perfringens* type D antitoxin (Lamb Dysentery Antiserum, Coopers Pitman Moore; Pulpy Kidney Antiserum, Hoechst).
- Supportive therapy (not glucose saline as hyperglycaemia occurs terminally) and warmth.
- Pain relief with Buscopan Compositum, (Boehinger Ingelheim), flunixin meglumine (Finadyne, Schering Plough) or pethidine.

Prevention

- Vaccination with a multivalent clostridial vaccine will give some protection against enterotoxaemia *Cl. perfringens* types B and C and tetanus. The immunity produced in goats is less satisfactory than that produced in sheep and there is some evidence that 4 in 1 vaccines give better protection than 7 or 8 in 1 vaccines. However any vaccine used should contain toxoids of *Cl. perfringens* types B, C and D and *Cl. tetani*, e.g. Lambivac (Hoechst). Six monthly boosters are necessary.
- Avoid digestive disturbances – overeating of concentrates, high concentrate diet with insufficient fibre, excessive grazing on lush grass etc. – and make any feed changes gradually.

NB Although generally considered a major disease of goats in the UK, difficulties in confirming the diagnosis mean that the true incidence is unknown. Any 'sudden death' is usually attributed by goatkeepers to enterotoxaemia so that other causes of sudden death, e.g. bacterial septicaemia or mesenteric torsion, are underdiagnosed. Even the finding of epsilon toxin in intestinal contents does *not* prove conclusively that death was caused by *Cl. perfringens* type D and *histological examination of the brain is essential for diagnosis.*

Urolithiasis

Urolithiasis (see Chapter 14) should be considered as a cause of colic in older male kids.

Visceral cysticercosis

Infecton with large numbers of *Cysticercus tenuicollis*, the metacestode of the canine tapeworm *Taenia hydatigena* occasionally causes acute disease in kids under 6 months because of damage to the liver parenchyma. Clinical signs include depression, anorexia, pyrexia, weight loss, abdominal discomfort and occasionally death due to acute haemorrhage.

Plant Poisoning

See Chapter 20.

Further reading

Enterotoxaemia

Baxendell, S. A. (1984) Enterotoxaemia of goats. *Proc. Univ. Sydney Post Grad. Comm. Vet. Sci.*, **73**, 557–560

16 Respiratory disease

Respiratory disease in goats is generally poorly researched worldwide. There is a paucity of information on the aetiology and frequency of respiratory disease in the UK, but it would appear to be relatively common, ranging from sudden death from peracute pneumonia to slight but persistent coughs and nasal discharges (Table 16.1).

Infectious diseases

Bacteria

- Pasteurellosis
- *Corynebacterium pyogenes*
- *Staphylococcal* spp.
- *Streptococcal* spp.
- *Haemophilus* spp.
- *Klebsiella pneumoniae*
- *Tuberculosis*

Mycoplasma

Viruses

- Herpes viruses, e.g. IBR (BHVI)
- Respiratory syncytial virus
- Parainfluenza virus 3
- CAE
- Pulmonary adenomatosis

Parasites

- *Muellerius capillaris*
- *Dictyocaulus filaria*
- Protostrongylus rufescens
- Hydatid cysts

Airway obstruction

- Foreign body
- Lymph node enlargement
- Tracheal collapse
- Tumour

Table 16.1 Differential diagnosis of respiratory diseases

(1) Nasal discharge
   Bilateral
      Rhinitis
         viral
         bacterial
         fungal ⎫
                  ⎬ unlikely, UK
         mycoplasmal ⎭
      Pneumonia (see cough)
      Dusty conditions

   Unilateral
      Sinisitis – *oestrus ovis?*
      Nasal tumour
      Foreign body

(2) Cough
   Pneumonia
      bacterial
      inhalation (drench, force feeding, dip, rhododendron poisoning)
      parasitic
      fungal (unlikely, UK)
   Allergic bronchitis
   Congestive cardiac failure
   Oesophageal obstruction
   Lymph node enlargement – lymphosarcoma, caseous lymphadenitis
   Tuberculosis

(3) Dyspnoea
   Primary respiratory disease
      bacterial pneumonia
      inhalation pneumonia
      chronic interstitial pneumonia (CAE)
      mycoplasma (*not* UK)
      pulmonary adenomatosis
      lung/nasal tumours
      tracheal collapse
   Heat stroke
   Poisoning
      cyanide (prunus family)
      nitrite/nitrate
      urea
      salt
      organophosphorus
   Anaemia
   Cardiac disease – congenital, acquired
   Bloat
   Selenium/vitamin E deficiency
   Hypocalcaemia
   Terminal stages of many disease conditions
   Trauma – thoracic injuries, diaphragmatic hernia

Inhalation pneumonia

Trauma

Heat stress

Allergic alveolitis

Neoplasia

- Primary/secondary lung tumours
- Intranasal tumours

Other conditions producing respiratory signs as part of a clinical syndrome

- Hypocalcaemia
- Poisoning – nitrite/nitrate; urea; organophosphorus
- Bloat
- Anaemia
- Selenium/vitamin E deficiency (white muscle disease)

Initial assessment

Consider:

- Individual or herd/flock problem.
- Possible exposure to infected animals – shows, brought in stock etc.
- Feeding, e.g. dusty hay; root crops etc.
- Housing – ventilation, building design.
- Vaccination.
- Overall level of coughing/sneezing in the building.

Clinical examination

- A thorough clinical examination should be made – temperature, pulse, respiratory rate, auscultation of the lungs – to localize lesions to the upper and lower respiratory tract.
- *Clinical signs of respiratory distress may arise from many conditions not directly related to the respiratory tract*, e.g. bloat, anaemia, hyperthermia, acidosis. *Hypocalcaemia* may present as an apparently excited, pyrexic and pneumonic goat.

Infectious disease

Respiratory disease may have have a multifactorial aetiology. Although several organisms known to produce severe respiratory disease in goats are absent from the UK, including the Mycoplasma responsible for contagious caprine pleuropneumonia (CCPP) and Peste des petits ruminants virus (PPRV), a number of infectious agents have been isolated from clinical cases or experimentally shown to produce disease in goats in the UK.

Bacteria

Pasteurellosis

Pasteurella haemolytica and *Pasteurella multocida* have been isolated from pneumonic lungs of goats.

P.haemolytica serotypes A1, A2 and A6 are the commonest isolates in the UK. The disease may be precipitated by stress, e.g. transport etc.

Clinical signs

* The disease syndrome of 'pasteurellosis' may involve other aetiological agents such as viruses or other bacteria and a wide variety of clinical signs ranging from occasional coughing to sudden death, but often an acute pneumonia, particularly in kids.
* Lethargic, anorexic, pyrexic.
* Tachypnoea, hyperpnoea, dyspnoea.
* Abnormal lung sounds – rales, rhonchi, noisy expiration.

Postmortem findings

* Exudative bronchopneumonia.
* Extensive consolidation of the lung.
* Fibrinous pleurisy.

Diagnosis

* Identification of *P.haemolytica* from a nasal or nasopharyngeal swab indicates that the organism is present *not* that the goat has pasteurellosis.
* Postmortem confirmation depends on bacteriology and histology of lung lesions.

- *Pasteurella multocida* has been shown to produce an atrophic rhinitis with nose bleeding, sneezing and nasal turbinate atrophy.

Other bacteria

Corynebacterium pyogenes, Staphylococcal spp., *Streptococcal* spp., *Haemophilius* spp. and *Klebsiella pneumoniae* among others have been isolated from infected goats.

Goats are susceptible to infection with *Mycoplasma bovis, M. tuberculosis* and *M. avium* (see Chapter 8).

Mycoplasma

Mycoplasmal infections have rarely been reported as causing respiratory disease in goats in the UK.

M.ovipneumoniae, which has been isolated from goats in Australia, Texas and the Sudan, has been isolated from sheep in the UK and may act as a predisposing agent for pasteurella infection.

M.capricolum, M.conjunctivae and *Acholeplasma oculi* have also been isolated from animals in the UK. Their role in respiratory disease is uncertain and they are discussed more fully in Chapter 19.

Outwith the UK, severe respiratory disease is produced by a number of mycoplasma e.g. *M.capripneumoniae* (F38 species), *M.mycoides* subspecies *capri, M.mycoides* subspecies *mycoides* (large colony type).

Viruses

The exact role of viruses in the aetiology of respiratory disease in goats in the UK is not known. Several viruses have been isolated from or shown serogically to be present in association with clinical disease.

Herpes viruses

Infectious bovine rhinotracheitis (IBR, BHV-1) virus has been isolated from goats with respiratory and ocular disease, although the goat may not be a natural host for the virus.

Caprine herpes virus type 1 (BHV-6) which causes vulvovaginitis and infertility in New Zealand and Australia does not appear to cause respiratory disease, but strains of caprine herpes virus in the USA caused severe systemic illness including dyspnoea in kids.

Respiratory syncytial virus (RSV)

Although RSV has been isolated from goats in the UK its role in respiratory disease is unclear. In the USA, RSV has been associated with nasolacrimal discharge, pyrexia and coughing.

Caprine arthritis encephalitis virus (CAE)

See Chapter 6. Some goats infected with CAE develop a progressive intestinal pneumonia characterized by a chronic cough and weight loss. Pneumonia may occasionally be the major presenting sign.

Pulmonary adenomatosis (Jaagsiekte)

A disease of sheep which has been transmitted experimentally to goats. There is a chronic progressive pneumonia with adenomatosis lesions of the lung alveoli.

Laboratory investigation

- Bacteriology – isolation of bacteria from nasal swabs does not confirm an organism as being responsible for disease, merely that it is present in the nasal passages; nasopharyngeal swabs are more useful.
- Virology – nasopharyngeal swabs can be used for virological examination.
- Paired serum samples 10–14 days apart may be of value.
- Postmortem examination
    histopathology
    bacteriology/virology etc.

Treatment of infectious respiratory disease

- Isolate affected animal(s) and carefully observe other animals for early signs of disease.
- Provide warm, draught free environment.
- Use antibiotics to control bacterial pneumonias or prevent secondary bacterial infection.
- Use non-steroidal anti-inflammatory agents such as flunixin meglumine (Finadyne, Kirby Warwick) 2 ml/45 kg i.v.
- Pasteurella vaccination – Pasteurella vaccines should contain *P.haemolytica* serotypes Al, A2 and A6 and all serotypes of *P.multocida*. Separate pasteurella and clostridial vaccines should be used rather than combined vaccines.

Control of infectious respiratory disease

- Strong well nourished kids will be less susceptible to respiratory infection.
- Avoid mixing different age groups in one air space.
- 'All-in-all-out' policy for batches of kids.
- Well ventilated draught free environment.

Parasites

Dictyocaulus filaria

- Infects both sheep and goats.
- Direct life cycle with larvae being passed in faeces.
- Found in the trachea and bronchi.
- Not often a major pathogen; respiratory signs most likely in the South of England during late summer/autumn following larval build-up on pasture during the summer.

Epidemiology

- Larvae overwinter on pasture.
- Carrier sheep perpetuate the infection.

Clinical signs

- Coughing, tachypnoea, naso-ocular discharge.
- Inappetence, weight loss.
- Secondary infection may result in pyrexia and dyspnoea but severe clinical parasitic bronchitis is rare.

Diagnosis

- Larvae in faeces after a Baerman or $ZnSO_4$ flotation.

Treatment

- Ivermectin, oxfendazole, fenbendazole, levamisole.

Muellerius capillaris

- Infects both sheep and goats; goats are more susceptible to disease.
- Indirect life cycle with slugs and snails ingesting the larvae and acting as intermediate hosts.
- Found in the alveolar ducts, small bronchioles, subpleural connective tissue and lung parenchyma.

Epidemiology

- Goats are infected during their first summer on pasture by eating intermediate hosts on herbage. Level of infection increases with age so that clinical disease is generally seen in adult goats over 3 years old.

Clinical signs

- Variable, ranging from mild cough to severe chronic cough and dyspnoea.

Diagnosis

- Larvae in faeces after Baerman or $ZnSO_4$ flotation.

Treatment

- Fenbendazole (30 mg/kg in single dose or 15 mg/kg daily for 3–5 days).
- Ivermectin (200–300 µg/kg).
- Neither drug is completely effective and will need repeating after about 3 weeks.

NB Levamisole, particularly in injectable form, may produce a hypersenisitivity reaction in the lungs due to the death of large numbers of *M.capillaris* and should thus be used with caution in any animals suspected of having heavy worm burdens.

Protostrongylus rufescens

- Not reported as pathogenic in the UK but reported as leading to secondary pneumonia and pleuritis in the USA.
- Found in the bronchioles.

Hydatid cysts

- A proportion of cysts reach the lungs and may produce respiratory signs particularly if a secondary pasteurellosis occurs.

Airway obstruction

Foreign bodies in the trachea or the oesophagus (see choke (see Chapter 14)) can result in coughing and signs of respiratory distress.

Lymph node enlargement in the neck can impede air flow (may be caused by caseous lymphadenitis).

Tracheal collapse has been recorded.

Tumour – thymomas or thymic involvement in multicentric lymphosarcoma may affect the respiratory or cardiovascular systems.

Inhalation pneumonia

May follow drenching, stomach tubing, etc. or *Rhododendron poisoning* (see Chapter 20) where vomiting results in inhalation of rumen contents.

Trauma

(1) *Throat* – injury to the throat from drenching gums or barbed plant material can result in cellulitis, pharyngitis and respiratory signs.
(2) *Thoracic injuries* – penetrating thoracic wounds, fractured ribs etc.
(3) *Diaphragmatic hernia.*

Heat stress

Goats being transported, confined in buildings or attending agricultural shows in hot weather will often show heat stress – excessive panting, increased heart rate, excessive thirst etc. Severe cases progress to respiratory and circulatory collapse, convulsions, coma and death.

Allergic alveolitis

Exposure to dusty conditions or feed may result in an allergic alveolitis with a chronic non-productive cough.

Treatment

- Remove from cause, damp hay; cough suppressants; clen-buterol (Ventipulmin injection/granules, Boehringer Ingelheim, 0.8 mcg/kg, i.e. 1.25 ml/50 kg i.m. or slow i.v. or 2.5 g/50 kg orally in feed twice daily).

Neoplasia

(1) *Primary and secondary lung tumours* are very rare.
(2) *Enzootic intranasal tumours* have been described in goats,with a serosanguinous nasal exudate, stertorous breathing and dyspnoea.

Other conditions producing respiratory signs as part of a clinical syndrome

(1) *Hypocalcaemia* (see Chapter 11) – may present as an apparently, excited, pyrexic and pneumonic goat. When in doubt give calcium and magnesium.
(2) *Poisoning*
   (a) *nitrite/nitrate poisoning*
   (b) *urea poisoning*
   (c) *organophosphorus poisoning*
(3) *Bloat* (see Chapter 14)
(4) *Anaemia* (see Chapter 17)
(5) *Selenium/vitamin E deficiency* (see Chapter 7) – kids with white muscle disease may show dyspnoea coughing and abnormal respiratory sounds.

Further reading

General

Harwood, D. G. (1989) Goat respiratory disease. *Goat Vet. Soc. J.*, **10** (2), 94–98
Martin, W. B. (1983) Respiratory diseases induced in small ruminants by viruses and mycoplasma. *Rev. Sci. Tech. Off. Int. Epiz.*, **2** (2), 311–334
McSporran, K. D. (1985) Pneumonia. *Proc. Course in Goat Husbandry and Medicine, Massey University*, November 1985, 123–125
Robinson, R. A. (1983) Respiratory disease of sheep and goats. *Vet. Clin. North Amer.: Large Animal Practice*, **5** (3), November 1983, 539–556

Mycoplasma

Jones, G. E. (1983) Mycoplasmas of sheep and goats. *Vet. Rec.*, **113**, 619–620
MacOwan, K. J. (1984) Mycoplasmosis of sheep and goats. *Goat Vet. Soc. J.*, **5** (2), 21–24

Lungworms

Lloyd, S. (1982) Control of parasites in goats. *Goat Vet. Soc. J.*, **3** (1), 2–6

17 Anaemia

Initial assessment
Clinical examination
Laboratory investigation
Treatment
Helminthiasis
Protozoal
Bacterial
Plant poisoning
External parasites
Trauma
Cow colostrum
Mineral deficiencies
Mineral poisoning
Protein deficiency
Chronic disease

Helminthiasis

- Haemonchosis
- Trichostrongylosis
- Fascioliasis

Protozoal

- Coccidiosis
- Eperythrozoonosis
- Sarcocystosis

Bacterial

- Leptospirosis

Plant poisoning

- Bracken (*Pteridium aquilinum*)
- Pyrrolizidine alkaloid poisoning
- Brassicas
- Onion

External parasites

- Sucking lice
- Keds

Trauma

Cow colostrum

Mineral deficiencies

- Copper (or molybdenum excess)
- Cobalt

Mineral excess

- Copper

Protein deficiency

- Primary or secondary

Chronic disease

- e.g. Johne's disease
- Tumour

Table 17.1 Anaemia

Cause of anaemia	PVC	Haemoglobin	Hypoproteinaemia	Bilirubin	Possible aetiology
Blood loss	Low	Low	Yes	Normal	Haemonchosis Trichostrongylosis Coccidiosis Lice Trauma
Haemolytic anaemia	Low	Low	No	High	Rape, kale or onion poisoning Copper poisoning Leptospirosis Eperythrozoonosis
Hepatic disease	Low or normal	Low or normal	Yes	High	Pyrrolizidine alkaloid poisoning
Hepatic disease + blood loss	Low	Low	Yes	High	Fascioliasis
Aplastic anaemia	Low	Low	No	High	Chronic inflammatory disease Protein deficiency Copper deficiency Cobalt deficiency
Protein loss	High or normal	High or normal	Yes	Normal	Coccidiosis Johne's disease Salmonellosis Trichostrongylosis

After Bennett (1983) *Vet. Clin. North Amer.: Large Animal Practice*, 5 (3), 511–524

Initial assessment

The preliminary history should consider:

- Individual or flock/herd problem.
- Grazing
    haemonchosis and fascioliasis common in certain areas
    access to poisonous plants.
- Feeding – Brassicas; onions; cow colostrum to kids.
- Trauma – accidents, fights or dog attacks, obstetric trauma.
- Anthelmintic treatment.

Clinical examination

Individual animals should be examined for signs of:

- Trauma/lacerations – may be internal haemorrhage without obvious external signs.
- External parasite infestations, e.g. sucking lice.
- Diarrhoea.
- Haemoglobinuria.
- Oedema – bottle jaw, ascites, ventral abdominal oedema.
- Many anaemic animals are also *hypoproteinaemic.*
- The mucous membranes should be carefully examined – pale or cyanotic or jaundiced.
- Cardiac rhythm may be altered with severe anaemia.

NB Jaundice is an uncommon sign in the goat even with severe hepatocellular damage but may occur (1) in *haemolytic diseases,* e.g. copper toxicity, leptospirosis, eperythrozoonosis and poisoning by Brassicas or onions where indirect (unconjugated) bilirubin levels are elevated or (2) following *bile duct obstruction* in fascioliasis or tumours where direct (conjugated) bilirubin levels are raised. In some cases of liver dysfunction, e.g. hepatitis or photosensitization both direct and indirect bilirubin levels may be elevated.

Laboratory investigation

(1) Blood samples – EDTA; serum; fixed smears. For normal haematological values, see Appendix 1.3.
Normcytic anaemia – infection, carcinomas, protein deficiency, cobalt deficiency, plant poisoning, acute fascioliasis.
Macrocytic anaemia – haemonchosis, recovery from trauma, eperythrozoonosis, subacute/chronic fascioliasis.
Microcytic anaemia – copper deficiency, chronic blood loss.
Examination of smears may show parasitized red blood cells (eperythrozoonosis) or abnormal shaped cells (poikilocytosis) associated with formation of a different type of haemoglobin (HbC).
(2) Faecal sample
   (a) Egg counts for haemonchosis and trichostrongylosis (see Chapter 13)
   (b) Egg counts for Fasciola if in 'fluke' area.
   Use sedimentation technique.

Treatment

(1) Specific therapy for particular disease.
(2) Supportive therapy to correct anaemia and hypoproteinaemia
    (a) Avoid stress – better to leave untreated than severely stress patient
    (b) Fluid replacement – lactated Ringer's solution 20–80 ml/kg depending on severity of fluid loss, slowly i.v.
    (c) Multivitamins/mineral preparation, e.g. Haemo 15 (Arnolds)
    (d) High protein diet
    (e) Blood transfusion – of value when animal is in shock following acute blood loss.
    Donor – CAE seronegative; take 10 ml/kg into collection bottle with 50–100 ml of 4% sodium citrate per 400 ml of blood.
    Recipient – give 10–20 ml/kg; avoid repeat transfusions; use adrenaline if transfusion reaction occurs. Blood can be given i.v. into the jugular or cephalic vein or more rapidly in kids intraperitoneally. An immediate improvement should be evident following i.v. transfusion and within 12–14 hours of peritoneal administration.

Helminthiasis

Haemonchosis

(See gastrointestinal parasitism, Chapter 13).

Severe anaemia and hypoproteinaemia may be produced very rapidly, before loss of condition is observed and a kid may be found dead. In less severe infections, death may result from chronic anaemia.

Diagnosis

- Anaemia/hypoproteinaemia.
- Abomasal contents reddish/black with 'barber pole' worms in large numbers.
- Faecal egg counts.

NB Suspect resistance to benzimadazole anthelmintics or underdosing (*weigh* animals) where goats have been regularly wormed.

Trichostrongylosis

(See gastrointestinal parasitism, Chapter 13).

Anaemia generally present as part of a clinical syndrome involving diarrhoea, weight loss, unthriftiness and hypoproteinaemia.

Diagnosis

- Anaemia/hypoproteinaemia.
- Egg counts.

Fascioliasis

See Chapter 8.

Generally chronic condition in goats, resulting in hypoproteinaemia and anaemia.

Diagnosis

- Anaemia/hypoproteinaemia.
- Faecal egg counts.
- Postmortem findings.

Protozoal

Coccidiosis

See Chapter 13.

Haemorrhage in the intestine may result in anaemia and hypoproteinaemia.

Diagnosis

- History .
- Clinical signs .
- Faecal oocyst counts .
- Postmortem findings.

Eperythrozoonosis

As *Eperythrozoon ovis* occurs in the UK and may infect goats, it should be considered as a remote possible cause of anaemia.

Babasiosis and anaplasmosis

Infect goats outwith the UK.

Sarcocystosis

See Chapter 2.

Bacterial

Leptospirosis

Goats do not appear to act as primary reservoirs of leptospiras, infection occurring spasmodically from contact with the organism in their environment or from carrier animals of other species.

Infection is generally poorly documented worldwide with the serovar *pomona* the commonest reported. Serological surveys in New Zealand have shown the serovars *bratislava* and *ballum* and *copenhagi* to predominate followed by *pomona, hardjo, tarassovi* and *australis*, but despite serological evidence of widespread exposure to leptospira species there was little evidence of active infection. No serological surveys of goats in the UK have been carried out.

Most animals exposed to leptospira do not develop clinical disease but, outwith the UK, sporadic reports of acute disease have been recorded. Severely affected animals are pyrexic and dyspnoeic with anaemia, haemoglobinuria and occasionally jaundice as a result of intravascular haemolysis. In goats, abortion is reported to occur only following septicaemia in acute infections, although in sheep the serovars *hardjo, pomona, ballum* and *bratislava* have been implicated in late term abortions, still births and the birth of weak lambs in the UK without other clinical signs of disease. *Hardjo* infection in sheep has been shown to produce an agalactia similar to that seen in cows, with soft udders, return to milk in 3–4 days and starvation of lambs if not hand reared. *Hardjo* has also been recovered from the brains of young lambs showing meningitis.

Plant poisoning

See Chapter 20.

Bracken (*Pteridium aquilinum*)

Goats seem less susceptible to bracken poisoning than sheep but prolonged grazing of the plant may result in an acute haemorrhagic syndrome or blood loss due to tumours in the bladder or intestine.

Pyrrolizidine alkaloids

e.g. *ragwort poisoning* (qv) results in haemorrhages following liver damage.

Brassicas

Prolonged feeding of kale and other Brassicas such as rape, cabbage, brussels sprouts and swede tops in large quantities results in haemolytic anaemia as a result of the conversion of s-methyl cysteine sulphoxide (SMCO) to dimethyl disulphide that destroys red blood cells.

Clinical signs

- Lethargy, inappetence, depressed milk yield.
- Anaemia, haemoglobinuria, jaundice.
- Pyrexia, tachypnoea.
- Diarrhoea.
- Death usually occurs in 24–48 hours.

Treatment

- Remove kale from diet.
- Treat anaemia.

Onions

Can be fed over long period without signs of poisoning but in large amounts produce haemolytic anaemia.

External parasites

Sucking lice

See Chapter 10.

Keds

Can also affect goats and produce anaemia.

Trauma

Chronic blood loss from internal or external wounds will result in anaemia.

Cow colostrum

Feeding bovine colostrum to kids may produce a haemolytic syndrome similar to that seen in lambs. Affected kids have severe anaemia and sometimes jaundice. The PCV declines to below normal by 7 days after birth and below 10% within 2 weeks, when clinical signs will be noticed. Initially lethargy and failure to feed, progressing to collapse and death.

Laboratory findings
- Direct Coombs' test demonstrates bovine IgG on erythrocytes.

Postmortem findings
- Extreme pallor, very watery blood; creamy appearance to bone marrow.

Treatment
- Blood transfusion (qv), corticosteroids, antibiotics and supportive therapy. Treat any other kids which have received the same batch of colostrum.

Mineral deficiencies

Copper deficiency (see Chapter 5)

May occur alone or in combination with cobalt deficiency. Anaemia occurs as a result of poor iron absorption with a resultant deficiency in haemoglobin synthesis and a microcytic, hypochromic anaemia.

Cobalt deficiency (see Chapter 8)

Results initially in normocytic, normochromic anaemia, often with haemoglobin and erythrocyte levels within the normal range because of haemoconcentration. Later there may be marked poikilocytosis and macrocytic anaemia with polychromasia.

Mineral poisoning

Copper poisoning

See Chapter 14. Results in an acute haemolytic crisis which occurs with sudden release of copper into the bloodstream when maximum hepatic levels are exceeded.

Protein deficiency

Primary protein deficiency due to malnutrition and secondary protein deficiency due to disease, e.g. Johne's disease may both result in anaemia.

Chronic disease

Chronic disease states, e.g. Johne's disease (qv) or alimentary tumours, may result in anaemia through blood loss or secondary protein deficiencies.

Further reading

Bennett, D. G. (1983) Anaemia and hypoproteinaemia. *Vet. Clin. North Amer.: Large Animal Practice*, **5** (3), November 1983, 511–524

18 Sudden death

Kids

Hypothermia/hypoglycaemia
Abomasal bloat
Ruminal bloat
Mesenteric torsion
Disbudding meningoencephalitis
Anaphylactic shock
Plant poisoning
Chemical poisoning
White muscle disease
Septicaemia
Coccidiosis
Enterotoxaemia
Listeriosis
Pasteurellosis
Haemonchosis
Salmonellosis

Adults

Ruminal bloat
Acidosis (ruminal impaction)
Trauma
Cold stress
Anaphylactic shock
Plant poisoning
Chemical poisoning
Hypomagnesaemia
Transit tetany
Gangrenous mastitis
Enterotoxaemia
Listeriosis
Pasteurellosis
Haemonchosis
Acute fascioliasis
Anthrax
Blackleg
Malignant oedema
Black disease
Botulism

Genuine 'sudden death' is rare in animals which are inspected
regularly.

Initial assessment

The preliminary history may play a major role in deciding the cause of death.

- Individual or group of animals involved.
- Recent introduction or movement of animal(s) involved.
- Age of animal, pregnant/non-pregnant, stage of lactation.
- Feeding – recent changes; access to feed etc., artificial rearing of kids, milk or milk replacer.
- Vaccination.
- Known disease status.
- Signs of ill health.

   Consider:

- Weather.
- Season of year.

Examination of carcase

- Position of body – posibility of trauma or electrocution.
- Signs of struggling? – terminal convulsions.
- Condition of body
   emaciated/good condition
   bloat
   discharges from orifices.

Postmortem examination

A thorough, prompt postmortem examination should be carried out. Delay will result in decomposition and reduce the chances of a successful outcome. Some causes of sudden death, e.g. some poisons, hypomagnesaemia, produce no obvious post-mortem changes.

Sudden death in kids

Non-infectious causes

Kids regularly die after short periods of abdominal pain or as result of trauma, e.g. strangulation in haynets.

   (1) Hypothermia/hypoglycaemia – see Chapter 5

(2) Abomasal bloat ⎫
(3) Ruminal bloat ⎬ – see Chapter 15
(4) Mesenteric torsion ⎭
(5) Disbudding meningoencephalitis – see Chapter 11
(6) Trauma
(7) Anaphylactic shock – it is commonly believed that goats are more likely than other species to suffer anaphylactic shock following repeated injections, particularly of procaine penicillin but also local anaesthetics and occasionally clostridial vaccines.
(8) Plant poisoning – see Chapter 20
Plant poisons may produce no obvious pathological changes, so that evidence of consumption or leaves in the forestomachs may provide vital information.
(9) Chemical poisoning – uncommon
Copper poisoning – see Chapter 14
Arsenic, lead (qv) and other metal poisonings produce acute or chronic illness, but occasionally present as sudden death.
Organophosphorus insecticides produce no obvious gross lesions at postmortem.
(10) White muscle disease – Chapter 7

Infectious causes

(1) Septicaemia, e.g. Pasteurella, streptococci
(2) Coccidiosis – see Chapter 13
(3) Enterotoxaemia (*Clostridium perfringens* type D) – see Chapter 15
(4) Listeriosis – see Chapter 11
(5) Pasteurellosis – see Chapter 16
(6) Haemonchosis – see Chapter 13
(7) Salmonellosis – see Chapter 13

Sudden death in adult goats

Non-infectious causes

(1) Ruminal bloat – see Chapter 14
(2) Acidosis (ruminal impaction) – see Chapter 14
(3) Trauma
(4) Cold stress – Angoras and Cashmere goats shorn in inclement weather without adequate shelter or nutrition
(5) Anaphylactic shock – see Sudden death in kids
(6) Plant poisoning – see Sudden death in kids

(7) Chemical poisoning – see Sudden death in kids
(8) Hypomagnesaemia – see Chapter 11
(9) Transit tetany – see Chapter 11

Infectious causes

(1) Gangrenous mastitis – see Chapter 12
(2) Enterotoxaemia (*Clostridium perfringens* type D) – see Chapter 15
(3) Listeriosis – see Chapter 11
(4) Pasteurellosis – see Chapter 16
(5) Haemonchosis – see Chapter 13
(6) Acute fascioliasis – see Chapter 8
(7) *Anthrax* – rare; peracute form may produce death in 1–2 hours. Acute cases may show pyrexia, tremor, dyspnoea and mucosal congestion. After death, dark unclotted blood discharges from nostrils, mouth, anus and vulva. Carcase undergoes rapid decomposition and there is absence of rigor mortis.

Diagnosis

● Blood smears from an ear vein should be air dried, fixed with heat and stained with polychrome methylene blue to show *Bacillus anthracis* rods with purple staining reaction of capsule.

If anthrax is suspected, the carcase should not be opened until the disease has been proved absent. If a postmortem has been carried out inadvertently there will be evidence of widespread haemorrhage and a grossly enlarged spleen.

(8) *Black leg* – rare; goats appear less susceptible than sheep.

Aetiology

● Acute infection by *Clostridium chauveoi (type B)* spores which enter by skin wounds or via the vulva and vagina at kidding or occasionally via the intestines and settle in muscle masses of the hind quarters, shoulder or lumbar areas. Bruising in these areas provides the anaerobic environment suitable for germination of spores.

Clinical signs

● Generally found dead, often a characteristic position with the affected limb stuck out stiffly and gas and oedema at the affected site.

- Decomposition and bloating occur rapidly and there may be blood from the nostrils and anus.

(9) *Malignant oedema* – acute anaerobic wound infection caused by *Clostridium septicum* (*chauvoci* type A) or other clostridial organisms; goats appear less susceptible than sheep.

Clinical signs

- Death occurs within 12–24 hours of first appearance of clinical signs; affected areas are swollen with emphysema, erythema and extensive frothy exudate from the wound.

(10) *Black disease (infectious necrotic hepatitis)* – rare; acute toxaemia caused by combined infection with the liver fluke, *Fasciola hepatica* (qv) and *Clostridium oedematiens* type B. Animals generally found dead with blood-stained froth from nostrils. Decomposition occurs rapidly. Postmortem shows dark subcutaneous tissue, blood-stained fluid in body cavities and a dark liver with scattered necrotic areas. In fluke areas, routine clostridial vaccination should include *Cl. oedematiens* type B toxin.

(11) *Botulism* – Ingestion of botulism toxin, produced by *Cl. botulinum*, in food has occasionally been reported to cause an acute onset paralysis or sudden death.

Further reading

King, J. M. (1983) Sudden death in sheep and goats. *Vet. Clin. North Amer.: Large Animal Practice*, **5** (3), November 1983, 701–710

19 Eye disease

Infectious keratoconjunctivitis
Foreign body
Trauma
Entropion
Photosensitization
Blindness

Keratoconjunctivitis

Infectious keratoconjunctivitis ('Pink eye', contagious ophthalmia)
Foreign body
Trauma
Entropion
Photosensitization

Infectious keratoconjunctivitis ('pink eye', contagious ophthalmia

Acute contagious disease characterized by inflammation of the conjunctiva and cornea in one or both eyes.

Aetiology

- The causal agents of the disease are still unclear, it is probable that several agents are involved.
- Predisposing factors include dusty hay, wind, bright sunlight and dust; overcrowding; long grass; flies.

Mycoplasma

There is strong evidence that *M.conjunctivae* is a major causal agent of keratoconjunctivitis in the UK.

Ureaplasma, Mycoplasma ovipneumoniae, Mycoplasma arginini and *Acholeplasma oculi* have also been isolated from keratoconjunctivitis in sheep and goats but their role in natural disease remains debatable. Predisposing factors such as wind or dust probably play an important part.

Rickettsia

Chlamydia psittaci produces keratoconjunctivitis in both sheep and goats. There may be abortions (see Chapter 2) occurring in the same herd/flock and polyarthritis in kids (see Chapter 7).

Rickettsia conjunctivae is reportedly a common cause of the disease in sheep and possibly goats outwith the UK, although in goats only a mild conjunctivitis is produced. It is probable that many cases attributed to this organism were in fact produced by *Mycoplasma* spp.

Bacteria

Bacteria probably act as secondary invaders where the primary damage is produced by smaller organisms, increasing the severity of the condition.

Branhamella ovis is commonly isolated from sheep with affected eyes.

Moraxella spp. may also be involved.

Listeria monocytogenes (see Chapter 11) may also cause keratoconjunctivitis as part of a syndrome involving neurological signs and/or abortion. Individual goats occasionally only show the ocular lesions – conjunctivitis, nystagmus, hypopyon and endophthalmitis.

Viruses

Infectious bovine rhinotracheitis (IBR) can cause a mucopurulent conjunctivitis in goats.

Transmission

- Flies and lice are possible vectors for the disease.
- Carrier goats exist for *Mycoplasma* spp. and *C. psittaci* and can thus introduce the disease into a new herd; carriers continue the disease within a herd and as immunity is poor individual goats may suffer repeated infection.
- Contact at shows will facilitate spread between herds.
- Close contact at feeding or even at grass will spread the disease within a herd.
- Cross infection occurs between sheep and goats.

Clinical signs

- Herd/flock problem as very infectious; Angoras may be more severely affected than dairy breeds; older goats may be more severely affected, following previous exposure.
- Conjunctivitis with marked hyperaemia, excessive lacrimation and blepharospasm so animals stand with affected eyes closed.
- Later corneal opacity and vascularization; corneal ulceration in severe cases with a purulent ocular discharge and possible rupture of the anterior chamber of the eye.
- Vision is affected in severe cases so animals may have difficulty feeding and lose condition.
- Cloudiness of cornea may persist for several weeks.

Diagnosis:

- Clinical signs as herd/flock outbreak.
- Swab *early* cases – vigorously swab conjunctivae and cornea
  (1) submit dry or in Stuart's medium for bacteriology
  (2) place in mycoplasma transport medium
  (3) place in chlamydia transport medium.
- Scrapings of everted conjunctiva can be placed on a slide, fixed in methanol and stained with Giemsa or examined using fluorescent antibody techniques for Mycoplasma or Chlamydia.
- Blood samples for chlamydia serology.

Treatment

- Topical tetracycline ointments daily for 5–6 days together with long-acting tetracycline injections intramuscularly, are generally effective if started early in the course of the disease.
- Long-acting tetracycline injections can be used prophylactically in the rest of the herd.

NB Treatment will not eliminate the organism in all cases, so carrier animals will remain to perpetuate the infection.

- Severely affected animals should be penned separately in dark surroundings with easy access to food and water.
- With severe corneal ulceration, third eyelid flaps can be used to protect the cornea.

Foreign body

Foreign bodies, such as seeds, shavings, etc. will result in severe conjunctivitis and possible corneal ulceration if untreated.

Foreign bodies may lodge behind the third eyelid and will need careful removal with the goat securely held. Sedation and/or the use of a topical anaesthetic such as 0.5% proparacaine (Ophthaine, Squibb) is advisable. After removal of the foreign body, treatment is as for infectious keratoconjunctivitis.

Trauma

The cornea of goats is commonly traumatized, often by stalks of hay or straw; overlarge tags on the ears of Angora kids may irritate the eye and the eye will also be damaged when entropion is present. Treatment involves correcting or removing the cause of the trauma then treating the resultant conjunctivitis or corneal damage.

Entropion

Entropion has been reported as an occasional congenital condition in all breeds of dairy goats and Angoras, but is uncommon in the UK. Because it is an heriditable defect, possible carriers, especially male goats, should be identified wherever possible. Surgical correction of the defect can be simply carried out using similar techniques to those used in the dog. Alternatively, the lower eyelid can be everted with skin sutures or by the subconjunctival injection of liquid paraffin or long-acting penicillin – the initial bleb produces immediate reversal of the entropion, followed by a degree of fibrosis which often prevents recurrence.

Acquired entropion can arise following trauma and scar formation.

Secondary bacterial infection may occur where chronic irritation of the cornea has been present for some time and should be treated with topical ophthalmic antibiotic ointments.

Photosensitization (see Chapter 10)

Photosensitization from whatever cause will affect the head resulting in swelling of unpigmented skin of the muzzle, drooping ears, swollen eyelids and ocular lesions, i.e. conjunctivitis, keratitis, excessive lacrimation, corneal oedema, blepharospasm and photophobia.

Affected animals should be removed from exposure to sunlight and any possible photosensitizing substance.

NB   *Cobalt deficiency (Pine)* (see Chapter 8) and *iodine toxicity* (see Chapter 5) can produce excessive lacrimation which might by confused with keratoconjunctivitis.

Blindness

Blindness is an uncomon presenting sign in goats, usually occurring in conjunction with other neurological signs (see

Chapter 11) or severe keratoconjunctivitis. The following conditions should be considered in apparently blind goats:

- Keratoconjunctivitis.
- Cerebrocortical necrosis.
- Pregnancy toxaemia.
- Pituitary abscess syndrome.
- Cerebral abscess.
- Coenurosis cerebralis (gid).
- Caprine arthritis encephalitis virus.
- Listerosis.
- Poisoning
    lead
    plant, e.g. rape
    rafoxanide.
- Focal symmetrical encephalomalacia.
- Scrapie.
- Louping ill.

Further reading

General

Baxendell, S. A. (1984) Caprine ophthalmology. *Proc. Univ. Sydney Post. Grad. Comm. Vet. Sci.*, **73** 235–237

Moore, C. P. and Whitley, R. D. (1984) Ophthalmic diseases of small domestic ruminants. *Vet. Clin. North Amer.: Large Animal Practice*, **6** 3, November 1984, 641–665

Wyman, M. (1983) Eye disease of sheep and goats. *Vet. Clin. North Amer.: Large Animal Practice*, **5** (3), November 1983, 657–676

Keratoconjunctivitis

Hosie, B. O. (1989) Infectious keratoconjunctivitis in sheep and goats. *Vet. Ann*, **29**, 93–97

Greig, A. (1990) Keratoconjunctivitis. *Goat Vet. Soc. J.*, **11**, (1), 7–8

Mycoplasma

Jones, G. E. (1983) Mycoplasma of sheep and goats. *Vet. Rec.*, **113**, 619–620

MacOwan, K. J. (1984) Mycoplasmoses of sheep and goats. *Goat Vet. Soc. J.*, **5** (2), 21–24

20 Plant poisoning

Goats, being of an inquisitive nature and of browsing habit, commonly consume poisonous plants. However, many goats seem able to consume small quantities of potentially harmful plants without ill effect, particularly when the rumen is full of other foodstuffs and there are very few well documented cases of plant poisoning occurring in goats in the UK. The rumen provides a significant protection from plant poisons for the goat when compared to monogastric animals. Thus moderate levels of oxalates, as found in sugar beet tops or rhubarb can be metabolized in the rumen and glycosidic steroidal alkaloids as found in solanaceous plants such as green pototoes and tomatoes can be safely hydrolysed. Most cases of poisoning are caused by garden shrubs, in particular rhododendrons, azaleas and laurels. It seems safest to assume that all evergreen shrubs are poisonous and to keep goat and plants well separated.

Many plants cause an *immediate poisoning,* e.g. yew, rhododendron. Some plants cause *delayed poisoning* as well as immediate poisoning, e.g. ragwort, St Johns wort etc.

Some plants are equally toxic when fed dry in hay, e.g. ragwort. Some plants are harmless when fresh but poisonous when dry and wilted, e.g. leaves of the *Prunus* family.

In addition to the plants listed in Table 20.1, British Goat Society publications list the following as being dangerous to goats at least under certain circumstances:

Mayweed, Old man's beard or Traveller's joy, Charlock, Bryony, Woody nightshade or Bittersweet, Deadly nightshade, Honeysuckle, Fool's parsley, Buttercup, Anemone, Lesser celandine, bulbs and their leaves, e.g. daffodil, tulip, aconite etc., Walnut and Spindle berry.

Some of the plants listed e.g. Walnut, are generally safe when eaten in small amounts but large quantities should not be given to stall fed goats.

Public health considerations

The excretion in milk of toxins from poisonous plants is unlikely in the UK, at least at high enough levels to provide a human health hazard. However, certain plant toxins, e.g. bracken toxins and carcinogens and pyrrolizidine alkaloids are known to be excreted in goats' milk and the possibility of affecting humans should always be considered, particularly as a particular goat's milk may be consumed by a limited number of people over a long period.

Table 20.1 Clinical signs of plant poisoning

Diarrhoea	Photosensitization	Vomiting
Hemlock	Ragwort	Rhododendron
Oak (young leaves)	St John's wort	Azalea
Wild arum	Buckwheat	
Castor seed (in foodstuffs)	Bog asphodel	*Goitre and still birth*
Foxglove		
Water dropwort	*Sudden death*	Brassica spp.
Box		Linseed
Potato (green)	Yew	Some clovers
Rhododendron	Laurel	
Linseed	Linseed	*Oestrus*
	Foxglove	
	Water dropwort	Some clovers
Constipation	*Frothy bloat*	*Stomatitis*
Oak (acorns and old leaves)	Legumes, e.g. rapidly	Giant hogweed
Ragwort	growing lucerne	Cuckoo pint
Linseed		
	Anaemia	
Nervous signs	Rape	
Ragwort	Kale	
Horsetails		
Hemlock	*Haemorrhage*	
Water dropwort	Bracken	
Potato		
Black nightshade	*Discoloured urine*	
Male fern		
Rhododendron	(a) Haematuria	
Laburnum	Bracken	
Rape	Oak	
Rhubarb	(b) Haemaglobinuria	
Common sorrel	Rape	
Sugar beet tops	Kale	
Prunns family	Cabbage	
	Brussels sprouts	

* Adapted from Spratling, R. *In Practice*, March 1980, 22.

Treatment of plant poisoning

Advice to owners:

- Separate the goat from the plant – it may be possible to actually remove the plant material from the goat's mouth.
- Keep the goat walking slowly so that it does not settle and start cudding.

- Give large quantities of strong tea (do not attempt to dose a vomiting animal). The tannic acid in the tea will precipitate many alkaloids and salts of heavy metals and will also have a useful stimulant effect.

NB Poisoning by acorns is due to their high tannic acid content – tea should not be given in cases of acorn poisoning.
Strong coffee will also have a stimulant effect.

- Large doses of liquid paraffin are also commonly used as a first aid remedy.
- Treat shock.
- If possible identify the source of poisoning.
- Give demulcents, e.g. a mixture of eggs, sugar and milk to soothe and relieve irritation of the stomach linings.

Veterinary treatment

- In most cases there is no specific antidote to the toxic principle involved in the poisoning and first aid should be continued together with symptomatic treatments, e.g. spasmolytics, intravenous fluids, oral laxatives, B vitamins and antibiotics if there is a danger of inhaling vomit.
- Rumenotomy should be considered to remove plant material, particularly if this can be done before clinical signs of poisoning have developed.

Specific plant poisoning

Rhododendron poisoning (rhododendron, azalea, kalma species)

Aetiology

- Commonest plant poison of goats in the UK, from browsing on the living shrubs and eating discarded prunings.
- Toxic principle is an andromedotoxin together with a glucoside arbutin.

Clinical signs

- Appear about 6 hours after ingestion of leaves.
- Lethargy, anorexia.
- Salivation, repeated swallowing.
- Abdominal pain.
- Vomiting.

- Ruminal bloat.
- Recumbency and death.
- Inhalation pneumonia may occur secondarily to the vomiting.

Postmortem findings

- No characteristic lesions.

Treatment

- Symptomatic and supportive therapy.
- Spasmolytics, B vitamins, antibiotics, analgesics.

Oxalate poisoning

Aetiology

- Ingestion of plants containing oxalic acid or its salts, e.g. Sugar beet tops, Mangold tops, Rhubarb leaves, Docks (*Rumex* spp.) and Wood sorrel (*Oxalis acetosella*).
- Goats can detoxify large amounts of ingested oxalates, so poisoning is only likely to arise if *large* amounts are eaten over a short period. Oxalates combine with blood calcium to produce insoluble calcium oxalate and severe *hypocalcaemia*.

Clinical signs

- Depression, inappetence.
- Muscular tremors, ataxia, staggering.
- Dyspnoea.
- Paralysis, recumbency and death.
- May present as sudden death.

Postmortem findings

- Calcium oxalate crystals in kidneys and urinary tract.
- Hyperaemia of the lungs; scattered haemorrhages.

Confirmation of diagnosis

- Oxalate can be detected in kidneys and rumen contents.

Treatment

- Calcium borogluconate.
- Provided treatment is early and kidney damage has not occurred there is rapid response to treatment.

NB (1) In castrated male goats, the urethra may become blocked by calcium oxalate crystals – this association of sugar beet tops with urolithiasis has led to the common misconception among goatkeepers that sugar beet pulp should not be fed to male goats.

(2) *Ethylene glycol (antifreeze)* poisoning results in increased salivation, ataxia, staggering, seizures, recumbency and death. Metabolites of ethylene glycol, e.g. glycolic acid formed by the liver are responsible for metabolic acidosis and hyperosmolality. Glycolic acid is excreted or further converted to oxalic acid with formation of oxalate cystals and signs of oxalate poisoning.

Diagnosis

- Ethylene glycol in rumen contents.
- Glycolic acid in urine serum or ocular fluid.

Photosensitization
See Chapter 10.

Prunus family poisoning (cyanide poisoning)
Aetiology

- The leaves of the *Prunus* family, e.g. Cherry, laurel, peach, plum, contain a cyanogenic glycoside amygdalin which is converted into hydrogen cyanide in crushed and wilted plants. Thus dried leaves are more dangerous than fresh leaves.

Clinical signs

- Sudden death.
- Dyspnoea.
- Muscular tremors, dilated pupils, ataxia, convulsions.
- Mucous membranes bright red.

Postmortem findings

- Blood bright red.
- Bitter almond smell of rumen contents.

Confirmation of diagnosis

- Cyanide estimation on rumen contents or blood (preserve with 1% sodium fluoride).

Treatment

- Rumenotomy.
- 1% sodium nitrite 25 mg/kg i.v. - induces the formation of methaemoglobin to which hydrocyanic acid is preferentially bound – followed by 25% sodium thiosulphate 1.25 g/kg i.v. which combines with hydrocyanic acid to form non-toxic thiocyanate.

Nitrate/nitrate poisoning

Aetiology

- Nitrates occur in many plants, e.g. Mangolds, Sugar beet tops and Rape. When excess accumulation of nitrate occurs, the plant may be toxic to ruminants. Poisoning is uncommon in the UK but in the USA and Australia may be caused by consumption of weed species which accumulate nitrite.

  In the rumen nitrates are converted to nitrite, which is absorbed and combines with haemoglobin in the blood to form methaemoglobin preventing the uptake of oxygen and resulting in *hypoxia.*

Clinical signs

- Depression.
- Abdominal pain, diarrhoea.
- Dyspnoea, convulsions, tachycardia.
- Ataxia, incoordination, coma and death.

Postmortem findings

- Chocolate coloured blood, petechiation of mucous membranes.

Confirmation of diagnosis

- Diphenylamine test on clear body fluids (urine, serum, CSF, aqueous humour).
- Nitrite estimation in blood or urine.
- Methaemoglobin estimation (stabilize sample in pH 6.6. phosphate buffer).

Treatment

- Adrenalin or etamiphylline camsylate (millophylline, Arnolds) i.v.

- Methylene blue, about 10 ml of 2% aqueous solution i.v. Repeat if necessary after 6–8 hours.

Kale poisoning
Haemolytic anaemia
See Chapter 17.

Goitre
See Chapter 9.

Ragwort poisoning

- Goats demonstrate an apparent tolerance to ragwort but are susceptible if enough is consumed over a long period (a total plant intake in excess of 100% of body weight may be required for toxicity to occur).

Aetiology

- Pyrrolizidine alkaloids contained in the plant are hepatotoxic. Poisoning can occur from the fresh plant or hay or silage.

Clinical signs

- Depression, inappetence, emaciation.
- Incoordination.
- Jaundice, anaemia.
- Hepatic neurotoxicity, coma, death.

Postmortem findings

- Enlarged cirrhotic liver.
- Petechial haemorrhages in the digestive tract.
- Spongy degeneration of brain and spinal cord.

Treatment

- None.

Plants affecting milk

The following plants are reported to affect milk (Cooper, M. R. and Johnson, A. W., 1984) but of course many also have for more serious affects.

Reduction in milk yield

Monkshood	Alder buckthorn	Buckthorn
Onion and garlic	Ash	Castor oil plant
Beet	Ivy	Sorrel
White bryony	Henbane	Water betony
Fat hen	St John's wort	Potato, green
Cowbane	Laburnum	Yew
Ergot	Mercury	Clover
Meadow saffron	Poppy	Hemlock
Bracken	Hawthorn	Oak
Cypress	Buttercup	Hounds tongue
Radish	Bluebell	Rhododendron
Horsetail		

Plants that can taint milk

Fool's parsley	Sweet clover
Onion and garlic	Mint
Beet	Wood sorrel
Turnip	Pea
Shepherd's purse	Bracken
Compositae spp.	Oak
Hemlock	Buttercup
Cress	Radish
Horsetail	Potato, green
Ivy	Yew
Henbane	Laburnum
Birdsfoot trefoil	

Further reading

Boermans, H. J., Ruegg, P. L. and Leach, M. (1988) Ethylene glycol toxicosis in a Pygmy goat. *JAVMA*, **193** (6), 694–696

Clarke, E. G. C. (1975) *Poisoning in Veterinary Practice*. The Association of the British Pharmaceutical Industry, London

Cooper, M. R. and Johnson, A. W. (1984) *Poisonous Plants in Britain*. MAFF Ref Book 161, HMSO, London

Jones, T. O. (1988) Nitrate/nitrite poisoning in cattle. *In Practice*, September 1988, 199–203

Mayer, S. (1990) Ragwort poison. *In Practice*, May 1990, 112

Seawright, A. A. (1984) Goats and poisonous plants. *Proc. Univ. Sydney Post. Grad. Comm. Vet. Sci.*, **73**, 544–547

Spratling, R. (1980) Is it plant poisoning? *In Practice*, March 1980, 22–31

21 Anaesthesia

Initial clinical examination

A routine clinical examination should be carried out in all animals to determine the degree of anaesthetic risk.

- General condition – fat cover, anaemia etc., age.
- Auscultation of heart and lungs:
  normal respiratory rate 15–20/minute
  normal pulse rate 70–95/minute.
- Accurate assessment of weight (*weigh* if necessary) – it is very easy to overdose if the estimation is inaccurate.

General anaesthesia

Preoperative considerations

Except for young kids, which are essentially monogastric, goats should be routinely starved for 12–24 hours preoperatively if elective surgery is being undertaken. Some authorities also recommend withholding water for a few hours. Longer periods of starvation may result in the rumen contents becoming more fluid with a greater likelihood of regurgitation occurring and may also predispose to the development of metabolic acidosis. Starvation means no food offered and no clean bedding, e.g. straw, either in the pen or in the vehicle used to bring a goat to the surgery.

Recumbency causes respiratory depression and hypoxaemia. The inspired gases should contain at least 30% oxygen (supply oxygen by mask if the goat is not intubated).

Premedication

Premedication before general anaesthesia is usually *not* necessary and often undesirable because of the increased time required for recovery.

To reduce the required dose of induction agent

Use of the following sedatives will reduce the dose of induction agent required (but also increase recovery time).

- Xylazine (Rompun, Bayer)
  0.05 mg/kg slowly intravenously or
  0.1 mg/kg intramuscularly.

Considerable problems and the deaths of many kids have been caused by overdosing with xylazine. Minute doses are required in young animals and it is very easy to overdose resulting, at least, in a very prolonged recovery. In kids, 0.025 mg/kg intramuscularly is probably the maximum safe dose. The standard 2% solution can be diluted and administered via an insulin syringe to enable more accurate dosing.

Angora goats are reported to require lower levels of the drug than dairy goats.

Xylazine is probably contraindicated in late pregnancy.

- Acepromazine maleate (ACP, C-Vet; Berkace, BK)
  0.05–0.10 mg/kg slowly intravenously.

Acepromazine is contraindicated in shocked animals because it produces a fall in blood pressure.

- Diazepam (Valium, Roche)
  0.25–0.10 mg/kg slowly intravenously.

Overdosage of sedatives

Overdosage of sedatives can be treated with:

- Doxapram hydrochloride (Dopram.V, Willows Francis)
  0.4 mg/kg intravenously.

In addition overdosage of xylazine can be treated with:

- Idazoxan
  0.05 mg/kg intravenously.

- Yohimbine
  0.1 mg/kg intravenously.

To reduce the flow of saliva

- Atropine
  0.4–0.7 mg/kg intramuscularly.

At this dose rate, atropine will reduce the flow of saliva but also render it more viscous, which may result in endotracheal tubes being blocked.

Most authorities do not recommend that atropine be given routinely as a premedication, although recognizing its use in situations where handling viscera may cause bradycardia and possibly cardiac arrest because of vagal inhibition.

Positioning of the goat during general anaesthesia

- Head down – allowing saliva to drain from the mouth.
- Neck placed over a sandbag.

- Hindquarters lowered – decreases pressure on diaphragm, reduces risk of regurgitation.

Injectable anaesthetic agents

(a) Barbiturates
- Pentobarbitone sodium 10–15 mg/kg intravenously.
- Thiopentone sodium 10–15 mg/kg intravenously.
- Methohexitone sodium 4 mg/kg of 2.5% solution intravenously.

In general the barbiturate drugs produce a marked respiratory depression, with delayed recovery if additional amounts are given to maintain anaesthesia. Regurgitation is particularly likely if thiopentone is used. Their use as sole anaesthetic agents is thus limited, but they are very useful induction agents before intubation and maintenance with gaseous anaesthesia.

Pentobarbitone is metabolized between three and four times faster in small ruminants than in dogs. Any commercial preparation containing propylene glycol should be avoided as haemolysis of red blood cells may be produced.

The short-acting barbiturates give a rapid, smooth induction. Giving half the calculated amount rapidly followed by the remainder over a 2-minute period may reduce the period of apnoea which occurs following rapid injection of the whole amount. Premedication with acepromazine or diazepam will reduce the barbiturate dose.

(b) Alphaxalone/alphadolone (Saffan, Coopers Pitman-Moore)

- Saffan 2.0–3.0 mg/kg slowly intravenously.

Saffan provides a reliable smooth induction agent in the goat with rapid recovery, minimal respiratory depression and less fetal depression than barbiturates, although a transient fall in blood pressure and heart rate occurs. Small goats, such as Angoras, require about 10 ml and larger dairy breeds up to 20 ml to produce a sufficient depth of anaesthesia for intubation. Kids presented for disbudding require between 1 and 2 ml intravenously. Laryngospasm and laryngeal oedema have been recorded in goats.

(c) Xylazine (Rompun, Bayer)/ketamine (Vetalar, Parke Davis & Co)

- Xylazine 0.1 mg/kg intramuscularly followed by

- Ketamine 10 mg/kg intramuscularly or 5 mg/kg intravenously.

Lower doses of xylazine (0.025 mg/kg) should be used in kids. Anaesthesia may be prolonged by incremental intramuscular doses of ketamine at 2.5–5.0 mg/kg or by use of gaseous anaesthetics such as halothane.

Ketamine has been used alone as an anaesthetic agent in goats but provides inadequate muscle relaxation for abdominal procedures.

(d) Diazepam (Valium, Roche)/ketamine (Vetalar, Parke Davis & Co)

- Diazepam 0.25–0.5 mg/kg intravenously, wait 2–3 minutes then
- Ketamine 4 mg/kg intravenously.

The lower level of diazepam is used in larger animals. This lower dose of ketamine will provide adequate time for intubation and maintenance on gaseous anaesthesia.

(e) Etorphine hydrochloride/acepromazine maleate (Large Animal Immobilon/Revivon, C.Vet)

- 0.5 ml/50kg intramuscularly or intravenously.

Large Animal Immobilon produces a reversible neuroleptanalgesia in goats as in other species and has been used for minor surgical procedures but there is reportedly a high mortality and morbidity rate.

Relapse due to recycling may occur, particularly if the intramuscular route of administration is used and can be countered by a further injection of Revivon.

The goat needs to be well restrained to avoid undue risk to the anaesthetist or assistant from an accidental self-injection of the drug and the relevant safety precautions should be carefully followed at all times.

(f) Etorphine hydrochloride/methotrimeprazine (Small Animal Immobilon/Revivon, C.Vet)

- 0.1 ml/kg intravenously.
- 0.05 ml/kg intramuscularly.

Small Animal Immobilon has been used in kids to provide anaesthesia for disbudding.

As with Large Animal Immobilon, safety procedures must be strictly followed.

(g) Propofol (Rapinovet, Coopers Pitman-Moore)

- 3 mg/kg slowly intravenously.

Propofol can be used to provide short duration anaesthesia with the advantage of rapid recovery.

Gaseous anaesthetic agents

(a) Halothane (Halothane, RMB; Fluothane, Coopers Pitman-Moore)

- Induction – gradual increase to 4%.
- Maintenance – 2%.

Halothane and oxygen is the most commonly used gaseous anaesthetic, providing excellent safe anaesthesia, either via mask for induction and maintenance of kids for disbudding, or for maintenance of older goats via endotracheal tube following induction by injection.

An oxygen flow of 11.0 ml/kg/minute is adequate.

Halothane hepatotoxicity has been reported (see Chapter 11).

(b) Methoxyflurane (Metofane, C.Vet)

Methoxyflurane will provide adequate anaesthesia in goats with a smooth recovery, but induction takes longer than with halothane and recovery is slower. Methoxyflurane is generally used for maintenance following induction with an injectable agent.

(c) Nitrous oxide

Nitrous oxide can be used during the induction of anaesthesia but should then be discontinued because it accumulates in the rumen and can potentiate ruminal tympany. When used for induction nitrous oxide should be 50% of the total gas flow.

Intubation

Intubation of goats can be performed with or without a long bladed laryngoscope. Endotracheal tubes about sizes 8–9 are generally suitable for adult goats. Comparatively, goats have a much smaller laryngeal opening than a dog and need relatively small tubes. An adequate depth of anaesthesia is essential for intubation. If a laryngoscope is not available, a technique of threading the tube through the larynx is relatively easy with experience. The goat is placed in lateral or dorsal recumbency and the tube inserted until the top touches the larynx, the larynx is then manipulated from the outside over the tube. A distinct click is usually felt as the tube passes into the laryngeal cartilages. The use of a wire stiffens in the tube may make the intubation easier.

Goats especially kids are prone to *laryngospasm* generally following regurgitation at the time of intubation. Spraying the cords with lignocaine will reduce the hazard. In an emergency, a tracheotomy may be necessary.

Hazards of general anaesthesia

1. Regurgitation

General anaesthesia (or deep sedation) can lead to passive regurgitation and aspiration of rumen contents.

The risk of regurgitation can be minimized by:

- Preoperative starvation.
- Correct positioning of the goat on the operating table. The thorax and neck should be raised if possible by tilting the table to lower the hindquarters, while the head is tilted downwards to allow free drainage of saliva.
- If problems arise during intubation, a cuffed tube in the oesophagus will help to protect the airway from regurgitation.
- If regurgitation occurs, the pharynx should be drained, the trachea sucked out and atropine administered if there is a danger of bronchospasm.

2. Salivation

Like all ruminants goats salivate copiously during anaesthesia and it is important that the saliva is allowed to drain freely from the mouth and not pool in the pharynx. Except for very short procedures the goat should be intubated with a cuffed inflated endotracheal tube.

3. Ruminal tympany

Ruminal tympany becomes progressively more important with the length of the operation as continuous gas production puts pressure on the diaphragm interfering with respiration and leading to hypoxia.

In elective surgery, preoperative starvation will reduce the risk of tympany or in non-elective surgery, rumen contents can be emptied by stomach tube, the contents kept at 37°C and then returned to the rumen postoperatively.

Removal of rumen contents by stomach tube may be possible if tympany occurs or the distension may be relieved by trocarization using a 14 or 16-gauge needle.

Depth of anaesthesia

No single reflex is reliable enough to be used on its own to assess the depth of anaesthesia. The assessment must be based on a combination of:

- Response to surgery – the anaesthetist should monitor the heart rate, pulse, respiratory rate, colour of mucous membranes, gingival perfusion time (normal 1–2 seconds) and muscle relaxation.
- Experience with the drug being used.
- Examination of a number of reflexes.

(a) *Jaw tension*: this decreases with an increasing depth of anaesthesia, but some tone persists even in deep anaesthesia. As the anaesthetic level lightens, swallowing or chewing movements can be elicited.

(b) *Eye rotation*: unlike cattle, eye rotation is *not* a useful method.

(c) *Pupils*: during surgical anaesthesia, the eye is normally *central* and the pupil moderately *constricted*. During both light and deep anaesthesia, the pupil is *dilated*.

(d) *Palpebral reflex*: this usually (but *not* always) disappears as surgical anaesthesia is obtained.

(e) *Limb withdrawal reflexes*: these are reduced during light anaesthesia with barbiturates or halothane and are generally absent under deep anaesthesia. However, they may persist if ketamine is used. Generally they are not as good an indicator of the depth of anaesthesia as in dogs and cats.

(f) *Corneal reflex*: this persists through all levels of anaesthesia.

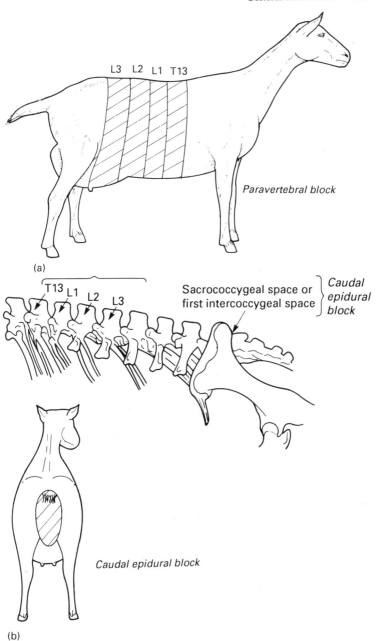

(a)

L3 L2 L1 T13

Paravertebral block

T13 L1 L2 L3

Sacrococcygeal space or
first intercoccygeal space

} *Caudal
epidural
block*

Caudal epidural block

(b)

Figure 21.1 (*a*) Paravertebral block; (*b*) Caudal epidural block

Local anaesthetics

Paravertebral anaesthesia

Use 5 ml of 1% lignocaine plus adrenaline – 2 ml above the intertransverse ligament and 3 ml below the ligament. The sites for injection can be palpated – inject 2 cm from the midline, the transverse process is 4–5 cm deep. Block nerves T13, L1, L2 and L3. Useful for Caesarian section or other abdominal surgery (Figure 21.1).

Caudal epidural anaesthesia

Inject 1–4 ml of 2% lignocaine through the sacrococcygeal space or first intercoccygeal space using a 19 g × 3.5 cm needle (Figure 21.1). This desensitizes the perineal area, tail and vagina and is useful for perineal surgery and some obstetrical conditions.

Local infiltration

Goats, particularly kids, are sensitive to the toxic effects of lignocaine and care must be taken not to exceed recommended doses, e.g. 30 ml of 2% solution in 45–68 kg (100–150 lb) goats and 40–50 ml in larger animals.

* Infiltration analgesia is useful for suturing wounds and as a line block for laparotomy where the anaesthetic is infiltrated along the line of the incision.
* *Inverted L block* – local anaesthetic is injected as an inverted L so as to block the nerves entering the operation site, creating an area of analgesia. The horizontal arm of the L is ventral to the transverse processes of the lumbar vertebrae and the vertical arm is posterior to the last rib (Figure 21.2). This technique avoids oedema of tissues, with subsequent delayed wound healing in the area of the incision.

Intravenous regional analgesia (IVRA)

IVRA is a technique for obtaining analgesia of the lower limb using 5 ml of 2% lignocaine injected via a 23 g needle into a superficial vein such as the medial radial vein in the fore leg and the lateral saphenous vein in the hind leg. The injection should be directed distally with pressure on the injection site to avoid a haematoma.

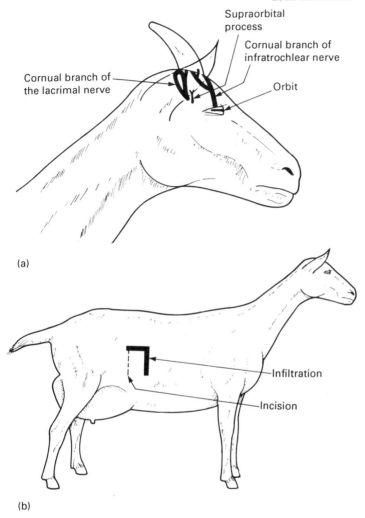

Supraorbital process

Cornual branch of infratrochlear nerve

Cornual branch of the lacrimal nerve

Orbit

(a)

Infiltration

Incision

(b)

Figure 21.2 (a) Local anaesthesia for dehorning; (b) inverted L block

A tourniquet is applied above the carpus or hock to localize the effect of the lignocaine and prevent its leakage into the circulation. A roll of bandage below the tourniquet on the lateral surface of the hock allows better occlusion of the blood vessels.

The onset of analgesia is about 5–10 minutes after injection and persists for as long as the tourniquet is left in place. The tourniquet should not be removed for at least 20 minutes and should not be left in place for more than 2 hours.

Dehorning

2–3 ml of 1% lignocaine at each of the following sites (see Figure 21.2):

- Cornual branch of lacrimal nerve is blocked as in the calf using the supraorbital process as a landmark.
- Cornual branch of the infratrochlear nerve is blocked dorsomedial to the eye close to the orbit.
- In kids, use a maximum of 1 ml on each side. General anaesthesia is safer and easier for routine disbudding (see Chapter 22).

NB Under most conditions, general anaesthesia is to be preferred to local anaesthesia for dehorning. For technique, see Chapter 22.

Further reading

Gray, P. R. and McDonell, W. M. (1986) Anaesthesia in goats and sheep. Part I, Local analgesia. *Comp. Cont. Ed. Pract. Vet.*, **8** (1), S33–S39
Gray, P. R. and McDonell, W. M. (1986) Anaesthesia in goats and sheep. Part II, General anaesthesia. *Comp. Cont. Ed. Pract. Vet.*, **8** (3), S127–S135
Taylor, P. (1980) Goat anaesthesia. *Goat Vet. Soc. J.*, **1**, 4–11

22 Disbudding and Dehorning

Disbudding and dehorning of goats can only be performed by a veterinary surgeon and the patient must be anaesthetized (Veterinary Surgeons Act 1966 as amended 1982).

Anatomy

- The horn bud in the kid is proportionately much bigger than in the calf.
- Two nerves supply the horn
  cornual branch of the lacrimal nerve.
  cornual branch of the infratrochlear nerve.

See Figure 21.2.

Disbudding of kids

Age

Kids should preferably be disbudded between 2 and 7 days of age, particularly males where horn growth is rapid.

The selection of anaesthetic agent for disbudding kids

See also Chapter 21.

Of all the domestic species, only kids are routinely anaesthetized so soon after parturition. Because they are alert and active and relatively large when compared to, say, an adult cat, it is easy for the veterinary surgeon to forget that they are dealing with a neonatal animal.

Kids are very sensitive to lignocaine like all neonates – analgesic doses are very close to toxic doses – and overdosage will result in lethargy, unwillingness to feed and even death. The toxic dose of lignocaine is about 10 mg/kg, i.e. 2 ml of 2% lignocaine for a 4 kg kid. Similarly only *minute* doses of xylazine are required – the ruminant dose is much less than that routinely used in the dog and cat and it is preferable to dilute the standard 2% solution.

At the surgery, induction and maintenance with halothane in oxygen by mask is simple, quick and safe and recovery is very rapid.

On the farm, Saffan (Cooper Pitman-Moore) is easy to administer, induction smooth and recovery quiet and relatively rapid. Depending on the size of the kid, 1 or 2 ml of Saffan is injected into the cephalic or jugular vein.

Equipment

Calf disbudding irons are quite adequate for disbudding small kids, provided they reach a satisfactory temperature. In this respect gas irons are probably better than electric irons. Dehorning irons, heated in a gas blow torch to 600°C are also suitable. A technique for disbudding kids using a tubular cutting edge has been described (Boyd, 1987).

NB Halothane/oxygen mixtures will support combustion of hair resulting in a rather singed kid – the anaesthetic mask should therefore be removed before a gas iron is applied.

Procedure

Clip the hair from around the horn bud. With larger buds clip off the tip of the buds with scissors or bone forceps if necessary. Apply the iron to the bud with an even action to ensure the whole bud tissue is destroyed – it is important to use a hot iron for the minimum time necessary to remove the bud. Excessive pressure or exposure may result in cortical necrosis, cerebral oedema and a brain damaged kid or even fracture of the skull. The whole bud is best removed, rather than just burnt around as this reduces the risk of infection.

Where the disbudding iron has a recessed head or the iron is not very hot, scraping the burnt out area with a scalpel blade and then briefly reapplying the iron ensures the tissue is destroyed. If the cauterized area is not large enough, a further ring of tissue can be removed with a scalpel blade or, even better, with an electric cautery knife. Several superficial vessels, especially the superficial temporal artery on the lateral side of the horn, may require re-cauterizing.

Finally the cauterized areas are sprayed with tetracycline spray, and antibiotics and tetanus antitoxin given.

Large buds are best removed with embryotomy wire as described in dehorning. Where kids are presented at about 3 or 4 weeks, it is extremely difficult to remove successfully all horn tissue with a calf disbudding iron – in these cases it may be best to wait for a few more weeks until the horn can be removed with wire.

Descenting of kids

Burning a semi-circular area caudomedially behind the horn buds will also remove the scent glands from the area, reducing to some extent buck odour. However, the presence of musk cells in other parts of the body and the habit of spraying urine means that even 'descented' males will still smell during the breeding season.

Dehorning

Horned goats, particularly when running with hornless animals, are often dominant within the herd. Dehorning can thus have profound psychological implications for the goat, involving loss of status, reduced milk yield or impaired fertility. Possible complications from surgery include sinusitis, myiasis and tetanus. After surgery, breathing can be seen to occur through the frontal sinuses and haemorrhage may occur down the nostrils. For these reasons the whole procedure should be carefully discussed with the owner and the timing of surgery arranged accordingly – surgery is best carried out in a dry, non-pregnant goat during the autumn, winter or early spring.

Removal of the horns exposes the openings into the frontal sinuses which extend into the hollow base of the horn. It is important that the openings are kept as clean as possible after surgery by treating regularly with antibiotic powders or sprays, feeding hay from the floor rather than a rack, and housing the goat in clean surroundings. The head is likely to remain tender for a month or more. Bandaging of the head is sometimes recommended or the holes can be covered in stockholm tar.

Anaesthesia

Local analgesia/sedation can be used (see Chapter 21), but a light general anaesthetic with halothane/oxygen or Saffan is preferable. No intubation is necessary if the operation is performed quickly on a starved animal.

Surgical technique

The hair is clipped from around the horns and the skin incised in a ring about 1 cm from the base of the horn. The horns are removed in turn with embryotomy wire working from the back of the horn forward and keeping the wire as low as possible to avoid leaving scars. Any haemorrhage should be controlled by cautery. Antibiotic and tetanus antitoxin should be given.

Descenting of adult goats

Descenting of polled, horned or disbudded adult males can be carried out under general anaesthesia.

A triangular skin flap is made with the base of the triangle approaching the caudal aspect of the head and the apex 3–4 cm in front of a line between the horns or polls (Figure 22.1). The

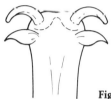

Figure 22.1 Incision line for scent gland removal

skin flap is separated from the underlying tissue and folded caudally to its base. The large scent glands, which generally lie within the borders of the triangle are exposed, grasped with forceps and removed with scissors or a scalpel blade, taking care to remove all glandular tissue. The skin flap is replaced with simple interrupted sutures. Antibiotic cover and tetanus antitoxin should be given.

Further reading

Anon (1984) Disbudding. *Goat Vet. Soc. J.*, **5** (2), 32–33

Boyd, J. (1987) Disbudding of goat kids. *Goat Vet. Soc. J.*, **8** (2), 77–78

Buttle *et al.* (1986) Disbudding and dehorning of goats. *In Practice*, March 1986, 63–65

Johnson, E. H. and Steward, T. (1984) Cosmetic descenting of adult goats. *Agri. Practice*, **5** (9), 16

Taylor, P. (1983) Goat anaesthesia. *Goat Vet. Soc. J.*, **1**, 4–11

Turner, A. S. and McIlwraith, C. W. (1982) Dehorning the mature goat. In *Techniques in Large Animal Surgery*, Lea and Febiger, Philadelphia, pp. 317–319

Appendix
The normal goat

(1) Physiological values

Temperature	38.6–40.6°C (average 39.3°C) (102–104°F)
Respiration	15–20/minute
Heart rate	70–95/minute
Rumination	1–1.5/minute

(2) Weight

Adult dairy doe	55–105 kg
buck	75–120 kg
Adult Angora doe	35–50 kg
buck	50–65 kg

(3) Haematology

	Unit	Range	Mean
Erythrocytes	$10^{12}/1$	7–21	14
PCA	ratio (1/1)	0.19–0.40	0.29
MCV	fl	15.0–39.0	21.0
Hb	g/dl	8.0–16.0	11.0
MCHC	g/dl	32.0–40.0	37.0
MCF (fragility)	% NaCl	0.60 (min)	
Viscosity (20°C)	centipoises	–	4.18
WBCT (clotting time)	min	–	4.5
Prothrombin time	s	–	11.1
Leucocytes	$10^{9}/1$	4.0–15.0	8.0
Neutrophils	%	40–50	42
	$10^{9}/1$	–	3.4

Lymphocytes	%	45–60	49
	$10^9/1$	–	3.9
Monocytes	%	2–6	3.0
	$10^9/1$	–	0.24
Eosinophils	%	2–10	6
	$10^9/1$	–	0.43
Basophils	%	0–1	<0.5
	$10^9/1$	–	0.03
Platelets	$10^9/1$	400–500	450
Blood volume	ml/kg	87.8–93.5	90.2

(4) Urinalysis

Specific gravity	1.015–1.050
pH	7.0–8.0
Colour	Yellow
Turbidity	Clear
Volume	10–40 ml/kg body weight/day

(5) Cerebrospinal fluid

Specific gravity	1.005
Colour	colourless
Total protein	0–39 mg/dl
Glucose	70 mg/dl
White blood cells	0–4 cells/µl

(6) Reproductive data

Breeding season (northern hemisphere):	September to March
Oestrus cycle (days)	: 21 (18–21)
Oestrus duration (hours)	: 32–96
Ovulation after start of oestrus (hours)	: 36–48
Age at puberty (months) male	: 4–5
female	: 4–5
Gestation period (days)	: 150 (145–154)
Semen Volume (ml)	: 0.5–1.5
Concentration (×10/ml)	: 1500–5000
Total sperm (×10)	: 750–7500
Good motility (%)	: 70–90
Normal morphology (%)	: 75–95

General references

Anatomy

Garrett, P. D. (1988) *Guide to Ruminal Anatomy Based on the Dissection of the Goat.* Iowa State University Press

Owen, N. L. (1977) *The Illustrated Standard of the Dairy Goat.* Dairy Goat Journal Publishing Corporation

Nutrition

Orskov, B. (1987) *The Feeding of Ruminants, Principles and Practice.* Chalcombe Publications

National Research Council (1981) *Nutrient Requirements of Goats, Nutrient Requirements of Domestic Animals.* Number 15, National Acadamy Press

British Goat Society. *Goat Feeding.* British Goat Society 34/36, Fore St., Bovey Tracey, Nr Newton Abbot, Devon TQ13 9AD

Management

Gall, C. (ed) (1981) *Goat Production.* Academic Press

Guss, S. B. (1977) *Management and Diseases of Dairy Goats.* Dairy Goat Journal Publishing Corporation

Mackenzie, D. (1980) *Goat Husbandry.* Faber and Faber

Mowlem, A. (1988) *Goat Farming.* Farming Press Books

Wilkinson, J. M. and Stark, B. A. (1987) *Commercial Goat Production.* BSP Professional and Books

Medicine and surgery

Baxendell, S. A. (1988) *The Diagnosis of the Diseases of Goats, Vade Mecum, Series B, No. 19, Univ. Sydney Post-Grad. Comm. Vet. Sci.*

Dunn, P. (1982) *The Goatkeepers Veterinary Book.* Farming Press Books

Goat Veterinary Society Journals, Matthews, J. (ed.). The Limes, Chalk Street, Rettendon Common, Chelmsford, Essex. CM3 8DA

Goats (1984) *Proc. Univ. Sydney Post-Grad. Comm. Vet. Sci.,* no. 73

Goat Health and Production (1990) *Proc. Univ. Sydney Post-Grad. Comm. Vet. Sco.,* No. 134

Howe, P. A. (1984) *Diseases of Goats, Vade Mecum No. 5, Univ. Sydney Post-Grad. Comm. Vet. Sci.*

Lloyd, S. (1982) Goat medicine and surgery. *Br. Vet. J.,* **138**, 70–85

Sheep and Goat Medicine (1983) *Vet. Clin. North Amer.: Large Animal Practice,* **5** (3), November 1983

Reproduction

Artificial Breeding in Sheep and Goats (1987) *Proc. Univ. Sydney Post-Grad. Comm. Vet. Sci.*, no. 96

Embryo Transfer Goats and Sheep (1989) *Proc. Univ. Sydney Post-Grad. Comm. Vet. Sci.*, No. 127

Evans, G. and Maxwell, W. M. C. (1987) *Salamon's Artificial Insemination of Sheep and Goats*. Butterworths, London

Haematology and biochemistry

Davies, D. M. and Sims, B. J. (1985) Welsh and Marches Goat Society survey to determine normal blood biochemistry and haematology in domestic goats. *Goat Vet. Soc. J.*, **6** (1), 38–42

Mews, A. and Mowlem, A. (1981) Normal haematological and biochemical values in the goat. *Goat. Vet. Soc. J.*, **2 (1), 30–31**

Index